Praise for *Vegan Love*

"Whether it's advice, great food, or a fashion find, Maya Gott~~f~~ ~~d i~~ ~~th~~e friend who's always there for you with compassion and a new way of looking at so~~r~~ to read this book and not feel like Maya has done you a solid
—Tracey Stewart, author of *Do* to *How Animals Live, and How*

"*Vegan Love* is a thoughtful, practical, timely guide to help vegans navigate the challenging terrain of finding rewarding relationships in a not-yet vegan world."
—Jonathan Balcombe, author of *What a Fish Knows*

"Maya Gottfried's delightful book *Vegan Love* offers great support for those seeking help in navigating romantic relationships while maintaining a cruelty-free lifestyle. Maya reveals that by staying true to our love for animals, we often inspire those around us to live more compassionately. Fun, honest, and informative, *Vegan Love* shows that our authenticity benefits both the animals and our relationships."
—Gene Baur, president and cofounder of Farm Sanctuary and author of *Farm Sanctuary* and *Living the Farm Sanctuary Life*

"Adopting a vegan lifestyle can cause tension with friends and relatives. This is especially true in love relationships. Vegans and those considering veganism will find support and answers to their questions in Maya Gottfried's book."
—Élise Desaulniers, author of *Cash Cow: Ten Myths about the Dairy Industry*

"Everything you need for falling in love, getting hitched, and living happily ever after vegan-style! Whether your soul mate is vegan, veg-curious, or not yet either, true love will find a way, and Maya Gottfried helps it along in this delightful book that draws on the experience of vegans who've found that romantic bliss can coexist beautifully with scrambled tofu and leafy greens."
—Victoria Moran, author and podcaster, *Main Street Vegan*

"Be gone vegan myths! Author Maya Gottfried shows us just how easy it is to integrate veganism into our everyday lives. *Vegan Love* offers great advice for new vegans and those new to the dating scene, too. A very powerful book."
—Stacey Wolf James, author of the wedding planning guide *Never Throw Rice at a Pisces*

"Practical, probing, and poignant, Maya Gottfried's latest book is a gift to all women who are embracing the vegan lifestyle. Filled with insight, guidance, and resources, this is a go-to book that sheds light on love and the vegan path. A wonderful contribution and a great read. Hats off to Maya!"
—Amy Hatkoff, author of *The Inner World of Farm Animals: Their Amazing Social, Emotional, and Intellectual Capacities*

vegan
love

vegan
love

DATING AND PARTNERING FOR THE CRUELTY-FREE GAL, WITH FASHION, MAKEUP & WEDDING TIPS

MAYA GOTTFRIED

ILLUSTRATED BY DAME DARCY

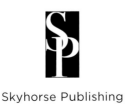

Skyhorse Publishing

Skyhorse Publishing books may be purchased in bulk at special discounts for sales promotion, corporate gifts, fund-raising, or educational purposes. Special editions can also be created to specifications. For details, contact the Special Sales Department, Skyhorse Publishing, 307 West 36th Street, 11th Floor, New York, NY 10018 or info@skyhorsepublishing.com.

Skyhorse® and Skyhorse Publishing® are registered trademarks of Skyhorse Publishing, Inc.®, a Delaware corporation.

Visit our website at www.skyhorsepublishing.com.

10 9 8 7 6 5 4 3 2 1

Library of Congress Cataloging-in-Publication Data is available on file.

Cover design by Jenny Zemanek
Cover illustrations by Dame Darcy

Print ISBN: 978–1–5107–1945–3
Ebook ISBN: 978–1–5107–1946–0

Printed in China

Contents

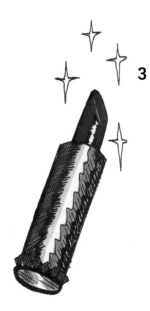

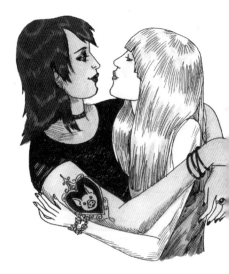

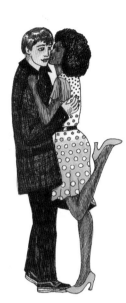

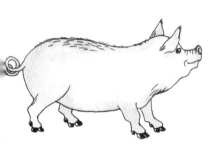

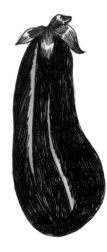

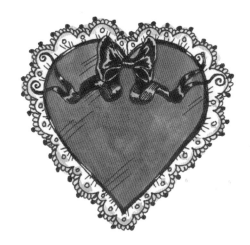

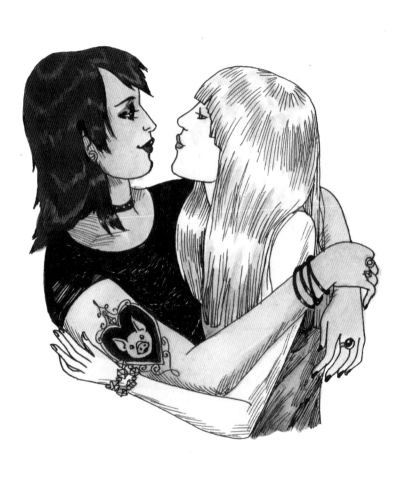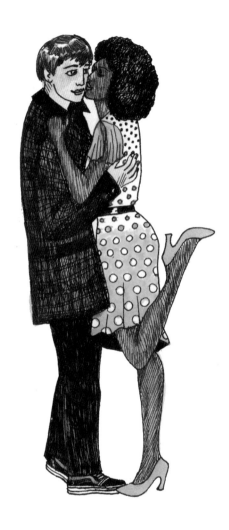

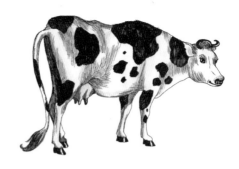

Out and Proud Vegan

I was in college when I first heard the term *vegan* and found out what it meant. I understood why someone would want to be a vegetarian, not eating animals, but I couldn't completely comprehend why a person would want to be a vegan, cutting all animal products out of his or her diet and life. A basic definition of *vegan* is refraining from consuming or using anything that comes from a non-human animal, whether those products appear in food, clothing, household items, or whatever else one might come across in life. That sounded like a pretty tall order to me.

I am an imperfect vegan despite trying my hardest to avoid all animal products, and my guess is that all other vegans are imperfect, too. I am certain that I've sat on a leather seat. I can say with confidence that despite believing a dish was vegan, at some point I was handed a meal with dairy in it at a restaurant, and sadly, I've run over insects with my car on the way into town. I do my best. When there's a choice to be made, I choose the compassionate route.

I've found that, despite my fears that going cruelty-free would be difficult, the world is generally vegan-friendly. If I'm in a clothing store, there are usually many more cotton and rayon (vegan) items than silk and wool (not vegan). When I've flown internationally, there has always been a vegan meal available on the plane (though I've needed to request it in advance). In foreign countries, I've consistently been able to find vegan food, whether in

Europe or Asia. Even when I order coffee at massive chains, I have options including soy and almond milk. Of course there have been challenging moments, and sometimes a little preparation (like packing my own food) has been required, but in the eight years since I went vegan, I have never been forced to eat an animal or gone without a meal.

When I made the commitment to go vegan at the age of thirty-five, I expected that a lot of challenges lay ahead of me. I was aware that my diet would change significantly. I dreaded the inevitable parting with non-vegan makeup. I felt fear as I surveyed my leather shoes, anticipating the day when I'd bid them adieu, and I experienced separation anxiety when I came across wool sweaters in my bureau. One thing I didn't take into consideration right away was how being vegan might impact my dating life. Soon, though, questions arose—more from curious friends and family than conjured up by my own mind. A close relative told me that as a vegan I would be difficult to date and suggested that it was not a smart path to take as a single woman in her thirties. A friend urged me not to tell dates about my cruelty-free lifestyle.

All of a sudden, I had to make decisions about when to tell someone I was dating that I was vegan and whether or not I could dine at a restaurant of that person's choosing. Should I put it in my online dating profile, save it for a phone conversation, or wait to gently explain it upon a first meeting?

This book's intention is to share with you my own and others' experiences of dating and partnering as vegans and help you find your own way. I believe you will discover, as I did, that it is much more of a stroll through a flower garden than a minefield.

I had always considered myself an "animal lover." Growing up in New York City, we had cats and dogs as companion animals in my home. I loved them and thought of them as part of the family. My heart would soar when I spotted wildlife, whether they were ducks on a pond or fish in a stream. However, I hadn't made the connection that the animals I was eating had also once been living beings with emotional lives, likes and dislikes, friends, family, and personality quirks just like the animals I lived with or saw scampering across the forest floor. For some reason, I completely separated my love for animals when I was putting food in my mouth.

Going vegan happened to me in one sudden, life-changing moment. I had gone vegetarian the previous year out of my love for animals and had been reading about factory farming and veganism for months. I had friends who were vegan. I saw it as a way to save lives on a daily basis by simply choosing not to eat certain foods or use particular products, and I wanted to take the plunge—yet I felt fear and doubt when it came to making the commitment. I had little faith that I could live my life without consuming animal products. I knew there were vegan lifestyle options a-plenty, but I had convinced myself that life would be significantly less enjoyable minus my eggs, cheese, and milk. That was my conundrum.

Of course there was also the panic caused by imagining a life of not being able to order anything I wanted in every single restaurant on the planet. People with severe nut allergies can't order just any item on a menu without risking death. Often kosher individuals dine only at certain restaurants, and those with celiac disease need to pick and choose their dishes carefully if they don't want to become sick. People exclude ingredients from their diets all the time for reasons ranging from saving their own lives to following religious traditions. Clearly, having limits on what I was able to eat was not the real problem.

I continued to read the evidence favoring a vegan diet. The facts are staggering.

According to the national farm animal rescue and advocacy organization Farm Sanctuary, 280 million hens laid 77.3 billion eggs in the United States in 2007. Male chicks won't grow to lay eggs and are therefore considered useless by the egg industry. About 260 million of them are killed each year, many being ground up while still alive. Ninety-five percent of egg-laying hens live in tiny cages granting them a space smaller than a sheet of letter-sized paper. In industrial farming facilities, chickens are crammed into cages and usually have their beaks cut with a hot blade at a young age to prevent them from pecking each other—behavior caused by their close confinement.

All of that so that I could eat a spinach and egg wrap in the morning.

But what about the milk in my coffee? According to Farm Sanctuary, in 2008 the number of cattle used in the production of milk in the United

States exceeded 9.3 million. These grand dames are confined in small spaces and continually impregnated (so that they will produce milk). The mama cows' calves are taken away, usually within hours of birth, while the mothers frequently bellow for their babies, experiencing horrific and visible emotional distress. Because the male calves will not grow to produce milk, they are usually raised for beef or slaughtered for veal at only a few months of age. Millions of them.

That's just the pain I caused at breakfast.

It finally hit me. I felt compassion and love for the animals, I wanted them to live happy and healthy lives, yet I felt a great disconnect from them—because I was hurting them. I could no longer deny the reality that the unnecessary choices I was making on a daily basis were causing pain to these beautiful, sentient, intelligent beings. It was as if I were a parent telling my children (the animals) that I loved them and then I was hurting them. Saying "I love you" doesn't erase the abuse. It doesn't stop the hurt. By going vegan, I was stopping the cruelty and letting the love shine through.

I listened to what I knew was true in my heart and acted accordingly. I simply believed that if I did what I knew to be right for me, everything else would work out. And it did.

When going vegan, I learned there is an abundance of vegan foods out there to be enjoyed. I didn't feel deprived; in fact, I tried many dishes I hadn't before, finding new favorites like tofu scramble and the Indian classic saag bhaji (a spiced spinach dish). Of course choosing to dine at a steak house probably would result in limited options, but plenty of restaurants offer a variety of delicious cruelty-free selections. Most importantly, avoiding certain foods was a small sacrifice to make for the sake of saving lives. I realized that forsaking ingredients painfully harvested from living, feeling beings was not difficult. I might have enjoyed the taste of a cheeseburger before I went vegan, but I don't need to eat them to live. The consumption of just one of those diner classics meant that a cow who might have enjoyed the sun on her back and the breeze against her face, a social animal with family and friends, had experienced an unnecessary death. Eating vegan just meant rethinking what I thought of as food, and by doing that I would save lives.

As soon as I eliminated the animal products from my diet, I instantly felt a connection with all beings that had previously been blocked. Whether it was a chicken living on a factory farm, or one of my companion cats purring on my lap, I experienced a deeper love for all animals. Perhaps that is not so surprising, but I also felt an increased compassion for human beings. I was no longer justifying violence, any violence. I had discovered that my life was sustainable without hurting others. Of course there are many unconscious ways we cause pain to other conscious beings. But by going vegan, I was making a choice that was significantly reducing my negative impact on others.

But then there's the issue of cravings. Some argue that a craving is our body telling us we need something. So if I craved milk or eggs, what would I do then? Our bodies often crave things that are not necessarily healthy: sugar, alcohol, and other controlled substances. My experience has been when I abstain from consuming what I crave, eventually the yearning for that substance disappears. When I first became vegan, I occasionally craved eggs, but I refrained from eating them, and at some point along the way I stopped desiring them.

I remember standing on a subway platform in New York City, soon after going vegan, and feeling a general lightness of spirit that I had not previously experienced. I knew I was consciously causing less suffering, and it changed my relationship with the world. I became aware that I had previously been subject to a subtle yet constant sense of guilt that was now gone. It was as though a wall had come down from around me. Somewhere in my subconscious, my entire being knew I was causing less pain, and I felt significantly better. It was a similar feeling to admitting to my dad, as a teenager, that I had used his credit card without his permission. Even though I justified purchasing those concert tickets in my seventeen-year-old mind, it was as if every part of me knew that it was wrong, and it haunted me until I told him. Then the veil lifted. The same guilty feeling disappeared when I went vegan. I just hadn't realized that it was there.

What I gained in losing hamburgers was emotional access to the billions of living beings I share the planet with. I felt a greatly increased sense of peace. I had lots of energy and was healthy.

Next, I veganized my lifestyle. In my closets sat many hundreds of dollars worth of leather handbags and shoes. In the top drawer of my bureau was a recently purchased pair of black leather gloves. Winter often found me cozily wrapped in wool scarves, and a family member had recently given me a sweater that flaunted a fur collar.

I don't know which was harder—the shoes or the handbags. They were just objects, but for some reason I was very attached to them. I reminded myself that cattle had died so that these accessories could be made. When thinking about going vegan, I had met and petted cows and steers at Farm Sanctuary's expansive shelter in Watkins Glen, New York, where hundreds of animals who have been rescued from the farming industry are cared for. I had experienced their incredible serenity, and their affection for bovine friends and human caretakers. I had even been nuzzled by a cow who had never met me before, freely offering me warmth despite having been previously hurt by members of my species. Still I clung onto these inanimate items made from the bodies of animals who I now considered my friends. Finally, knowing the truth in my mind, I ignored my more materialistic side and let go. I filled a bag with the shoes and got rid of them, giving some to a friend and dropping the rest off at a thrift shop. There was no justifiable reason that animals should suffer for the sake of my fashion sense.

I dreaded, in particular, letting go of one purple purse with gold detailing. I had spotted it in a local store and stalked it for months while the price remained too high for my modest budget. Finally, one day I strolled into the shop to discover the coveted leather satchel on sale for 50 percent off. I swiped my debit card and brought it home. When I went vegan, I balked at giving it away. Wasn't it divinely ordained that I should have that bag? Hardly. I don't think the powers above want me hauling dead bodies around. I packed it up along with the rest of the expensive handbags that I barely ever used and donated them to a community center.

Now my closets contain gorgeous cruelty-free shoes and handbags. I've learned that vegan designers take care of my every fashion-induced desire, and that animals don't need to suffer in the name of style, just as they don't need to suffer for my food. Now I get to walk around knowing that no one died for the sake of my vanity. Letting go of my non-vegan accessories was also an important reminder to me that some things are more important than possessions.

And then, just as I had finished veganizing my life, I was blindsided. A week after turning thirty-six, I found out I had cancer. Stage three colon and rectal cancers, to be specific. I was instantly launched into a completely different life than what I was used to. I left my job as a publicist at a respected New York City book publishing company within a week of the surprise diagnosis and embarked on a full-steam-ahead journey to save my life. My path to wellness included surgery and chemotherapy. I also incorporated complementary therapies such as restorative yoga, visualization, and acupuncture. I drank lots of vegetable juice. I was intent on doing everything I could in order to stay alive, and in my mind I would accept no other outcome. I was shocked but I was hopeful. Though there were horrible days of feeling overwhelmed by the side effects of chemotherapy, I maintained a positive attitude and focused on all of the love that surrounded me.

Many of my relationships with friends and family became stronger during this time. One of my favorite memories of those days was spending an evening camped out in bed eating takeout food with a friend while we watched a Duran Duran documentary, transfixed by the film like teenagers. With our busy grown-up lives, it had been hard to find space in our schedules for quality time together, but now my friends and I had a great excuse to just hang out and appreciate one another. I made myself vulnerable to the people around me and they reached out to help, even if it just meant sitting and keeping me company while I lay weakly in my small apartment, or coming with me on the subway when I went to the hospital. It was a difficult time with some very bright moments. When I was feeling depleted and sick, I still enjoyed the effects of my now regular meditation practice and the sunshine pouring through the window at the studio where I practiced yoga. In the end I recovered, but I realize how lucky I was. Others around me with similar positive attitudes lost their lives to the disease. It was during that year of treatments that I learned veganism not only saved the lives of animals, but it could help save my life, as well.

One evening, nauseous and weak from chemo, I went to a talk and book signing by the president and cofounder of Farm Sanctuary, Gene Baur. I got the opportunity to speak to Gene one-on-one for a few minutes at the small Brooklyn shop, and he mentioned a book titled *The China Study*, stressing the importance of its contributions in the area of nutrition. A little embarrassed that I hadn't heard of what was clearly an important entry in any vegan's library, I quickly purchased it. I read as I sat in the waiting room at Memorial Sloan-Kettering Cancer Center before my chemotherapy treatments, and when lying in bed at home, recovering from the harsh effects. Among the many revelations about the health benefits of a plant-based diet, the book presented undeniable evidence that being vegan could help prevent the growth of cancer; that the consumption of animal proteins did nothing less than facilitate the lethal disease's spread. Going vegan wasn't a cancer cure-all, but animal products undoubtedly helped cancer along.

Could I have been encouraging the growth of this disease inside me by what I had been eating all of those years? Though I had known before that as a vegan I could be as healthy as an omnivore, now I knew that veganism could make me healthier than those who consumed animals. Now not only did I stand strong in my new lifestyle for the sake of the animals, but I held onto it for my own life. I was already a devoted vegan, but after reading *The China Study*, I was certain that a plant-based diet was a crucial part of my path to good health. It turned out that what was best for the animals was also best for me.

And, by doing what was best for animals, and for my own good health, I was doing what was best for the planet. The farming of animals is incredibly destructive to the environment in a number of different ways. Massive amounts of manure are produced in the raising of animals for food. In fact, as reported by the United States Environmental Protection Agency (EPA), "a single dairy cow produces about 120 pounds of wet manure per day which is equivalent to the waste produced by 20–40 people." According to Farm Sanctuary, "Factory farms typically store animal waste in huge, open-air lagoons . . . which are prone to leaks and spills." In 2012, an Illinois pig farm spilled waste into a creek, killing more than 140,000 fish. The *Chicago Tribune* newspaper found that pollution from hog confinements killed at least 492,000 fish in Illinois from 2005 to 2014. In a report titled "Livestock's Long Shadow," The Food and Agriculture Organization of the United Nations

(FAO) states ". . . the livestock sector is a major stressor on many ecosystems and on the planet as a whole. Globally it is one of the largest sources of greenhouse gasses and one of the leading causal factors in the loss of biodiversity, while in developed and emerging countries it is perhaps the leading source of water pollution."

Even with life or death issues staring us in the face, and awareness that the planet is being destroyed, we can still be concerned about seemingly superficial lifestyle issues like, *What if my favorite perfume isn't vegan? What do I do then?* Given all of the above information, why wouldn't I be vegan? Because I couldn't continue to wear the same perfume?

As a vegan, I've been asked a lot of questions about shoes and sweaters and makeup. The truth is that these seemingly trivial items can be fun to indulge in. If they weren't available in vegan forms then I might be a little bummed out. Luckily, I don't have to fantasize about fancy footwear and lip color because there are so many vegan options to choose from. I can take the train from my upstate New York home into Manhattan and soon be surrounded by footwear options aplenty at vegan shop MooShoes (or buy online from my comfy couch). I can even walk into the local mall and have a wealth of vegan makeup products to choose from. I just need to do a little research online beforehand to confirm which are free from animal products.

More than one person showed concern for how a single gal like me would be able to date as a vegan. I still start to burn up when recalling warnings that being vegan might make dating difficult. It was as though someone suggested I not take life-saving medicine at a restaurant because it was a social faux pas. It was a no-brainer to me. I was going to be vegan no matter what. If someone had a problem with it, that was their problem. But the truth was, being vegan did have the potential to throw a possible partner for a loop. It didn't prevent me from dating, but there were some new considerations to keep in mind.

Dating as a vegan, I prioritized being true to myself and honest with those I dated. I didn't hide my veganism under a bushel—I let it shine. I also didn't pressure those I dated to share my way of living. I wrote in my profile at the dating website I used that I was vegan. When going on dates, I was open to going to non-vegan restaurants, as long as there was something I could eat.

The truth is that veganism didn't really come up in conversation that much on my dates. Mostly I was just trying to get to know the people I was going out with, finding out what they were interested in. One date enjoyed comedy so we chatted about the short film he was making while sitting at a café a few blocks from my Brooklyn apartment. Another person I went out with a few times was an opera singer whose day job was at the United Nations. We talked about the children's books I'd written over steamy beverages at a cute SoHo teahouse. I didn't speak too much at first about my ethical commitments, because our conversations often went in other directions. When questions did come up, I calmly shared with my date what I knew, passing on information that had helped me find my plant-based path. I discovered that by staying true to my love of animals and being honest, I avoided those who couldn't embrace my veganism and steered clear of dating disasters. I spoke from the "I" perspective (not telling them what they should do, but what I had experienced), and nobody argued with me. The truth is that I didn't run into one person who had a problem with my being vegan.

I had detailed why I didn't consume dairy to one tall, artistically talented crush of mine, an omnivore. In telling him, I explained that the cows are forcefully impregnated so that they will produce milk, and their calves are taken away from them. We left it at that and I didn't pressure him to go vegan. He had mentioned to me that friends of his family ran a small dairy farm. Originally he had told me he thought it was an ethical operation. A few weeks later, he said he had visited the farm and his friends who ran it. He had asked if they took the calves away from the mother cows. "They do," he said very seriously, clearly having taken in the gravity of that act. He had processed a very important piece of information—that cruelty is inherent in the farming process, even at small dairies. He may not have immediately become vegan, but because I was honest with him, he had the opportunity to see the truth for himself and is now conscious of the suffering in that industry—a big step. He became a good friend, and whenever we have gone out to dine, he's offered to eat vegetarian. I learned a truth, too: that we are better suited as friends than romantic partners. So by being honest, with him and with myself, everything worked out for the better in the end.

Being honest and truthful can be a little scary, but I've never regretted telling it like it is. Sometimes I feel a little bit like holding my breath when talking to an adamant omnivore about my vegan lifestyle, but no one I've dated has ever criticized or even questioned my commitment. If anything, they have been curious and shown admiration.

I never needed to, but had a date ever responded to my vegan values with antagonism, I like to think I would have put the kibosh on any potential relationship and deemed the scenario a no-go. Negativity toward something so important to me is not a trait I would tolerate in someone I was dating, and implementing that boundary didn't prevent me from meeting great potential partners. Overwhelmingly the response I experienced was positive. The disaster dates I did have had nothing to do with my being vegan.

I'm only one person, and there are a lot of vegans who are dating or in relationships. So in writing this book, I turned to them. To think that I have all of the answers would be silly. What I learned above all in interviewing these women and the people who love them is that there is a beautiful world out there for vegans who are looking for or living in relationships.

While researching the book, I heard no accounts of terribly uncomfortable dates during which someone was taken to task on their cruelty-free lifestyle. I was pleasantly surprised to be told no stories of someone needing to end a date early or exiting a relationship because they were disparaged for being vegan. In many cases, veganism was part of the bond one had with a partner—their love of animals becoming a place where they connected. For others, living with an omnivore was an opportunity to share compassionate qualities with a person who they loved, and they often saw their partner move toward a more cruelty-free lifestyle. Some people will let it be known right away that they don't want to date a vegan, and that makes it clear that they are probably not worth pursuing. Plenty of people out there embrace the vegan lifestyle, and I found there is no reason to waste one's time with someone who looks down on it. You may end up opting out of certain scenarios, like getting engaged to a butcher, but cutting out the cruelty doesn't mean forgoing a love life.

There are no rules when it comes to dating and partnering as a vegan gal, but there are many ladies who have traveled the path and found love by being true to themselves and honest with others. In being honest, one woman even found that someone who wouldn't date a vegan actually respected her choice of a cruelty-free lifestyle. Whether settling down in a long-term relationship or continuing to hop around the dating block, vegans I interviewed for this book have found peace and happiness by looking inside their hearts to realize their beliefs and needs and communicating those with others. Over and over again, the testimonies of vegans clearly lead to the conclusion that there is no conflict between a love for animals and a loving relationship. If anything, vegans who have stepped up to the dating plate and gone through the motions of introducing their lifestyles to new people have seen others grow in surprising ways, often going vegan themselves.

I've also included a wealth of information on makeup, fashion, and weddings. Dating and partnering isn't all about the practical, but material matters undeniably come into play. Let's face it: getting ready for a date has the potential to take as long as the date itself. Weddings often involve many months of planning. Whether your tastes are more casual, or you are a fan of the extravagant, I've provided tips, ideas, and resources to find what you are looking for, while cutting out the cruelty.

CHAPTER 1

The Dating Game: Looking For Love as a Vegan

Dating as a vegan brings with it a new set of questions and conundrums, concerns, and considerations. What I learned from my own experiences, and speaking with vegan women who are dating or in relationships, is that honesty is indeed the best policy. When I respect my own feelings and beliefs, and am truthful with others about who I am, I find the people who appreciate me and am able to let go of those who don't.

Above Average

Not long after I'd recovered from my cancer treatments, one of my lady friends and I chatted in a cozy bar on Manhattan's Lower East Side, exchanging dating tips and stories. It was a true girls' night out, complete with concert tickets to see a singer whose work I adored, Kristin Hersh, fronting her band, the Throwing Muses. My pal and I sat huddled in the amber glow of the dimly lit bar, comparing notes and confiding in each other. In the midst of talking, she advised, "Don't tell them you're vegan." In part I'd anticipated this remark, yet sat somewhat stumped.

The Language of Vegan Love

Throughout this book, some terms will come up that may be unfamiliar to you. Here are explanations of what they mean.

Cruelty-Free: In this book, I use the term *cruelty-free* to indicate that something does not involve harm to animals and is vegan. The cosmetics industry uses the term *cruelty-free* to indicate that a product was not tested on animals. However, in the case of cosmetics, these "cruelty-free" products may contain animal ingredients and therefore not be vegan.

Ethical Vegan: Someone who eschews animal products in the interest of helping animals, not only for health or environmental reasons.

Pescatarian: A person who eats fish or other seafood, but no land animals.

Plant-Based: The definition for this term varies depending on who is asked. As nearly all vegan foods are derived from plants, in this book I use the term *plant-based* to refer to food or a diet that is vegan.

Sanctuary: Sanctuaries are generally shelters providing high-quality care for rescued animals, usually with a great deal of land for the animals to roam. However, some organizations using the term *sanctuary* may not offer the high standards of those included in this book.

Vegan: Not eating or drinking any animal-derived ingredients, including (but not limited to) meat, dairy products, and eggs. In addition to food and beverages, vegans eschew animal products in other areas of their lives (such as clothing and makeup).

Vegetarian: A person who does not eat the bodies of any animals (including land animals and fish).

I've heard whispers among acquaintances that vegans are "high maintenance," "difficult," or "demanding." Advocates for omnivorous diets have peppered the media with comments implying that vegans are disrespectful of their dinner hosts and of traditions. There is a lot of fear-perpetuating propaganda out there.

My friend at the bar was concerned that by revealing my animal-product-free lifestyle, I might scare off prospective suitors. I worried, as she did, that the word *vegan* could trigger fear in the heart of the average man. But did I want to date the *average* man? The answer was *No, I didn't.* I wanted to date the above-average guy. And I told her that not only would I not hide my vegan lifestyle, but I would stand strong in my vegan boots. Perhaps I would even decide to date only other vegans. Veganism is a huge and bright light in my life, and I was not going to sweep it under the carpet for fear of remaining single. Since becoming vegan, I felt significantly better, both physically and spiritually. I was conscious that my daily decisions about what I consumed meant that there was less pain and suffering in the world. My involvement in activism fueled my sense of purpose—I wasn't just living my life for me anymore, but for other beings, as well. In becoming vegan, I had reached inside of me and realized what I truly yearned for: to be kinder to the animals I shared the planet with and not cause them pain. I had become vegan by living my truth. Was I really going to find love by living a lie?

It was a revelatory moment for me. I, like so many other single and seeking ladies, had been working to twist and contort myself into the perfect mold of the desirable date. Don't wear costume jewelry, don't put on too much makeup, don't dress in quirky clothing, don't tell them that you're vegan. I was finally fed up. I don't know what struck this faith in my heart that being true to myself was the answer, but I realized that I needed to pay attention to my own feelings and comfort levels—and not try so hard to fit a generic format that was rumored to be the ticket to love (and wasn't working for anyone I knew).

I didn't make it a rule to only date other vegans; I just promised myself I'd respect my own feelings and beliefs. I was not going to hide my vegan lifestyle, but instead pay attention to whether I was comfortable dating those who consumed animal products. If I wasn't, I wouldn't. If love is about honesty and being true to one's heart, wouldn't that include being honest about and true to one's love for animals? The question for me changed from whether or not someone could love me when I didn't eat animals, to whether or not I could love someone who did.

The answer was complex, certainly not black-and-white. However, what I found was that as soon as I put my foot down about being open, out, and unapologetic about my veganism, people started to respond in a very positive way.

I was subscribed to one online dating site with mixed feelings. I'm a big believer in serendipity when it comes to relationships, and I wasn't sure if that translated to the Internet. I was very clear in my profile that I was vegan, but I didn't indicate whether I would exclude omnivores from my dating pool. I heard from vegans, vegetarians, and omnivores alike.

I went on a date with someone who was vegan for health but not ethical reasons. He was creative, tall, smart, and funny. We met at a café in my Brooklyn neighborhood and talked over tea. He was a few years younger than me but I felt completely comfortable with the age difference. We agreed that we enjoyed our time together and made plans for a few nights later. I got all dolled up for the big night out, but before we met, I received a text from him, canceling due to a hefty hangover. I suggested he try seltzer next time. Although we ate similarly, there were some other connections missing. Eating alike didn't mean that we were compatible, and we went our separate ways.

The second person I went out with after committing to wear my veganism with pride was a good-looking and talented omnivore. He seemed very interested in and fascinated by my vegan lifestyle, activism, and general love of animals. We had a lovely tea date, and another at a museum devoted to Himalayan Asia. Despite our mutual enjoyment of these outings, it was not a love connection due to a lack of chemistry. I never even had to watch him eat something that I found offensive because we only met a couple of times. Once we decided not to take things further, he expressed his belief that I probably would not have liked his apartment as he had a cow-skin rug. He was right, but by staying true to my heart, I never had to see it in person.

Another fellow I interacted with on the dating website was, like me, a devoted vegan. We had even both spent time at Farm Sanctuary's shelter for rescued farm animals in Watkins Glen, New York. He was attractive and nice and considerate. He let me know that he worked at a successful company and lived outside of Boston, a city I enjoyed. But there was something missing. Although the common love for animals was present, and he seemed to be a kind, responsible, intelligent person, that little bit of magic just wasn't there.

My next romantic rendezvous almost didn't happen. My wariness of meeting people through the Internet led me to suspend my online dating account. Before I did, I heard from someone who the universe seemed to be urging me to connect with. A vegetarian (but not vegan) for many years longer than myself, there were no rational reasons why this date might go better than the others—only an instinctual sense to follow through. He had too many good qualities to mention and listed a number of bands in his profile that were favorites of mine as a teenager. Date #1 turned into dates #2, #3, #4, and more. We connected in many ways, a mutual love of animals being one of them. I loved classical music but didn't know much about the composers, while he had an encyclopedic knowledge of those works. I loved abstract expressionist art and he decorated his walls with paintings from that period. He loved cats and I had two. There was more that brought us together. We were a match, but not because I had created a checklist and he fit the bill; it was because of something deeper—an instinct, an internal voice, that pointed me in his direction. At the time of writing this, we have been together for almost five years, and the cats couldn't be happier.

I know someone who has been a vegan for many years and is happily in love with and married to someone who eats animal products. Another vegan who follows her path might have a life that looks much different.

What I learned was a simple, age-old lesson: by being open to what the universe brought me and letting go of situations that simply were not working, I was led to the best place for me.

Why Go Vegan?

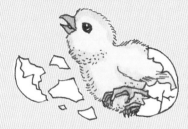

By committing to a vegan lifestyle, we save animals from suffering, but that's not the only compelling reason to make the switch. Cutting out the cruelty also helps the environment and allows us to live healthier lives.

For the Animals

Chickens

- Billions of chickens are slaughtered each year in the United States for their meat. The vast majority of these social and sensitive birds are held in deplorable conditions and bred to reach large, unhealthy sizes in a short amount of time—causing disease and early death.
- In the United States, 260 million male chicks are killed every year because they are considered useless by the egg industry, often being ground up alive.
- Hundreds of millions of chickens in the United States suffer a miserable life in tiny cages so that their eggs can be farmed.
- Because the overcrowding that chickens are subject to causes them to hurt one another with their beaks, young female chicks farmed to lay eggs are usually debeaked, having a portion of their beaks painfully removed.
- Chickens in the egg industry are often manipulated into an extra cycle of egg production by being denied food for as long as two weeks.

- Chickens who are no longer considered productive egg-layers are deemed "spent" and subject to an early death.

Turkeys

- Hundreds of millions of turkeys lose their lives in the United States every year so that they can be eaten. Many are killed for holiday meals, which could easily feature vegan options instead.
- Because they are bred to reach an abnormally large size, turkeys on factory farms can no longer reproduce naturally. Farmers use artificial insemination to breed them.
- Turkeys are inquisitive, social animals who enjoy walking in the grass and making friends with other birds and people. On factory farms, they are crowded together in huge buildings with only a tiny amount of space to live out their entire lives.
- Turkeys on factory farms live in horrible conditions and are closely confined, which they often react to by injuring one another with their beaks and toes. Because of this, they are usually debeaked and have portions of their toes removed at a young age.

Cows

- Cows in the dairy industry are forcibly impregnated repeatedly so that the mothers will produce milk. Their baby calves are taken away so that the milk is available for market instead. The mama cows express visible, overwhelming grief at the loss of their babies.
- Male calves taken from their mothers are generally either raised to be slaughtered for beef or killed at a very young age for veal.
- When separated from their mamas, calves become so upset that they often become sick, and according to Farm Sanctuary, "cry so much that their throats become raw."
- Most dairy cows spend their lives confined indoors, without the freedom to wander on the grass and graze or express their very social natures.

- Cows have been documented exhibiting tremendous fear, distress, and a strong desire to survive while awaiting slaughter. So prevalent is their panic and upset that some slaughterhouses are designed specifically to prevent animals from becoming aware of their impending death.

Pigs

- Pigs are complex beings, with high levels of intelligence, and strong emotional bonds to other pigs and humans who care for them.
- Pigs who are held on farms for breeding are generally confined in gestation crates—tight metal enclosures that are barely bigger than their bodies and too small for them to even turn around.
- Pigs held in gestation crates exhibit signs of extreme stress including biting the bars that surround them and chewing at the air.
- Piglets are taken from their mothers only weeks after birth before being sold for slaughter.
- The nonprofit organization Mercy for Animals released undercover footage that revealed workers on a farm hurling piglets across rooms and viciously throwing them into transport carts. They cut the youngsters' tails with dull pliers and threw injured and sick piglets into "gassing kill carts" to slowly suffocate from carbon dioxide.

Goats

- Goats are known for their playfulness and are often compared to dogs in their great affection for human companions.
- Goats who are farmed to be food generally lose their lives at a very young age, often being sent to slaughter at only three to five months old.
- Similar to cows in the dairy industry, baby goats (or "kids") are usually taken from their mothers immediately upon birth. The male kids are considered useless by the industry because they cannot bear children or produce milk, and are killed as infants.

Sheep

- Millions of sheep and lambs lose their lives in the United States every year, slaughtered for their meat.
- These sheep are generally held in horrible conditions and killed at young ages, never having the opportunity to enjoy the pleasures of running in the grass or lazing in the sun, as sheep at sanctuaries do.
- When farmed for their wool, sheep suffer terribly. Many are subjected to mulesing, which sees large areas of their skin cut from their backsides.
- Sheep raised for wool also experience painful and traumatic shearing.

For the Environment

- The Food and Agriculture Organization of the United Nations (FAO) states that animal agriculture is one of the largest sources of greenhouse gasses globally, a major factor in diminished biodiversity, and a leading source of water pollution.
- According to the United States Environmental Protection Agency (EPA), 1,799 gallons of water are required for one pound of beef.
- In the United States, 56 million acres of land are devoted to growing feed for animals.
- Animal agriculture creates vast amounts of manure. According to the EPA, factory-farmed animals in the United States produce approximately 500 million tons of manure per year. Without proper solutions for managing the excrement, it can cause significant damage to the environment. Pollution from pig-farming facilities killed nearly half a million fish in Illinois from 2005 to 2014.
- Noxious gases escaping farms' manure lagoons have been known to be fatal.

For You

- There is a great deal of scientific evidence that eating a vegan diet helps fend off various cancers, heart disease, type 2 diabetes, and obesity. It can also assist in managing Lyme disease and various digestive problems.

- Many who go vegan express feeling happier, healthier, and more connected to animals and humans alike.
- Vegans often report a significant increase in energy.
- Vegans can live knowing they are making decisions on a daily basis that reduce the suffering of others.
- Those who become vegan frequently report healthier skin and a newly glowing complexion.
- Being vegan connects us with the vast and supportive vegan community, offering the opportunity to connect with others based on core values.

Dating Stories: Are You Experienced?

Not every person you consider dating may be open to dating a vegan. But would you want to date someone who doesn't respect who you are? When the vegan women I interviewed were honest with others about their ethical lifestyles, letting unsupportive people fall away, they found dates and long-term partners who embraced their cruelty-free values. In being open about their compassion for animals, these women often found love with another human being.

When we go on a date with someone, that person has usually expressed some interest in us. This offers a great opportunity to put our best foot forward, and show that individual a glowing example of a happy, healthy, and kind vegan. Living by example can be a great form of advocacy.

Style Savvy Feline-Lover Meets Like-Minded Match
Jesse Oldham, Senior Director at an Animal Welfare Organization

When she isn't tending to her high-level job at one of the United States' most revered animal welfare organizations, Jesse Oldham can be found snuggling with her six cats, running the local food co-op's animal welfare committee, or scouring New York City's hottest used clothing shops for cruelty-free finds. Jesse currently lives with her boyfriend, also a devoted vegan, in Brooklyn, New York.

In addition to her professional interest in animals, Jesse is an expert on many animal-related topics, such as the care of feral cats and the vegan status of various cosmetics. She puts that knowledge to use by looking after homeless felines and educating others about vegan products. Even with all of her work to help animals, and her incredibly busy schedule, she manages to look glamorous, with elegant vegan makeup and playfully patterned dresses that show off her colorful tattoos.

Now vegan for more than twenty years, Jesse recalls her love of animals as a child: "I was one of those kids who would buy feeder goldfish from the pet store to save them." Jesse also had a "veg-epiphany" when she was young, while treating her family's companion dog for a wound: "I remember thinking [the wound] looked a lot like meat."

In addition to her natural love of animals, Jesse points to key influences that helped her down the vegan path as a young adult. "I was listening to punk music and reading fanzines like *Well Fed, Not Animal Dead* . . . so the concept of veganism kept popping up." She adds, "I think the saying that pushed me from vegetarian to vegan was, 'There's a veal calf in every glass of milk.'" This refers to the frequent farm practice of impregnating cows so that they produce milk and taking the newborn calves from their mothers to be slaughtered for veal.

Though Jesse is now comfortably settled in a committed relationship, she has plenty of experience playing the dating game. Before meeting her vegan match, she dated quite a few non-vegans. Jesse likes to let dates know about her cruelty-free lifestyle right away. She jokes with an example of outing herself to someone: "A) I have a lot of cats, and B) I'm vegan: if we want to proceed, we can proceed."

Because Jesse has found that omnivores often respond defensively to someone's claim of a vegan lifestyle, she suggests a gentle approach. "I try to do it as off-hand and low-key as possible . . ." For example, when planning a date at a restaurant with someone new, a few days prior she might say, "Oh, I'm vegan, you know, can I see the menu? I'm just going to double-check that I can eat here, if not, would you mind going here . . .?" This is a simple route to let the truth be known without tempting conflict.

Throughout her dating experiences, Jesse has found people to be generally respectful of her ethics concerning animals. Those who don't want to date a vegan have quickly stepped out of her way.

Though not a requirement for Jesse, having a vegan partner comes with major benefits. "I've certainly dated people who are not vegan in the past, but it is such a huge selling point to have somebody who you hope has essentially the same values as you." She appreciates not having to worry that her partner might want to purchase non-vegan products for their home, like a leather couch, or cleaning products that were tested on animals.

Jesse's kindness, combined with her honesty in dating, has landed her in a long-term relationship that doesn't challenge her deeply held vegan values. By being genuine and forthcoming with partners, Jesse has found someone who doesn't just tolerate her cruelty-free lifestyle, but embraces it.

Jesse encourages vegan women who are dating to steer clear of any person who ridicules them for their compassionate lifestyle. She also suggests broadening one's social circle. "There aren't that many vegan guys out there," she says, explaining that the community of vegan lesbians is not huge either. She recommends keeping one's options open and not being too quick to cross someone off the list of potential partners. Though Jesse eventually landed with a person who shares her cruelty-free lifestyle, many omnivores will be supportive of a partner's veganism. Often meat-eaters will move toward a plant-based diet when they become romantically involved with a vegan. By going on just one date with an omnivore, you may inspire them to test the vegan waters. If you find it too uncomfortable to be around someone who eats animals, you can follow in Jesse's footsteps and find a vegan to love.

Keeping Cruelty Off the Dinner Table
Cody Winchester, Works at a Health Center

Cody Winchester is a proud and very active vegan, having been involved in many animal rights causes during the two decades since she committed to a cruelty-free lifestyle. For her, having a long-term relationship with a meat-eater is not an option.

Cody's love and sense of responsibility for animals play a huge part in her life. She has organized animal rights protests and conferences, served as an adoption counselor at her local humane society, and been a wildlife rehabilitator. She is also on the board of directors for the Sanctuary and Safe Haven for Animals (SASHA) Farm, a rescue organization for farm animals in Michigan.

When it comes to dating, Cody has learned from experience. Previously married to an omnivore, she discovered that having a long-term partner who eats animals is not something she is willing to live with. "I was married for twenty-three years and my husband went vegetarian for two of those. He started eating meat again because he found it too hard . . . I had changed so much in all my beliefs during this time and we just grew apart," she says. Cody listened to her heart and realized she doesn't want to witness animal cruelty at the dinner table on a daily basis.

With this in mind, following her divorce Cody signed up for a dating service specifically for vegans and vegetarians—but didn't make a love connection. Now she looks for potential partners through other means. She makes a habit of telling her dates upon first meeting that she is vegan and that she can't sit across a table from them if they have an animal on their plate. "I believe in being up-front right off the bat, because if they are not even open to the idea, I don't want to waste his or my time." She adds, "I generally find men are interested in veganism and I try to explain to them my reasons and have always been respected for that." Cody is, however, open to dating omnivores who agree not to eat animals in front of her, keeping in mind that they may convert.

In continuing to date men who might become vegan, Cody's ethics have proven contagious. "I met a man a couple of years ago and he was a 'dog person.' Our first date was [at] a vegetarian restaurant and he became interested in my views. Three weeks in and he turned vegan all on his own."

Cody finds that because her omnivore dates are often interested in veganism, dating becomes an opportunity for education. When I ask her if anyone has not dated her, or ended a relationship with her because she is vegan, she plainly answers, "No."

For Cody, the process of a partner becoming vegan can be an exciting aspect of the relationship. "I think compassion for animals is very sexy; I loved watching my previous man holding a lamb for the first time and playing with baby pigs. I could see he was getting it!" she says.

Cody has taken on a number of roles with animal organizations, but her activism doesn't stop when it comes to dating. She has discovered that being honest about her beliefs and how she came to veganism is sometimes enough to inspire a partner to consume fewer animal products. She knows what she can and cannot tolerate and has moved forward from there. She doesn't keep her beliefs or lifestyle a secret for the sake of trying to find a mate, and in being forthcoming has seen a positive response in others, with their own compassion coming to the fore.

A Voice For the Animals Finds Love By Speaking Up
Jane Velez-Mitchell, Journalist
Donna Dennison, Works in the Film Industry

Jane Velez-Mitchell is a celebrated journalist who now stands in charge of her own online media outlet, *JaneUnChained*. Previously, she hosted her self-titled television show, *Jane Velez-Mitchell*, on CNN's HLN cable channel. A longtime vegan and activist, during her time at HLN, she featured an animal segment on her show each week, making her one of few media figures to bring animal rights issues to a national audience in the United States.

Today she works with romantic and business partner Donna Dennison to create *JaneUnChained*, producing videos on animal rights issues that are featured at various online outlets including the JaneUnChained.com website and numerous social networking platforms. Jane and Donna (known as "That Snarky Vegan Girl" on social media) use compelling videos to educate the public about animal cruelties and veganism. But Donna wasn't vegan when the two met.

The couple first crossed paths at a Santa Monica, California, restaurant when Donna walked in to meet a group of women that included Jane.

"She had just come back from Turks and Caicos and I had never met her, and she's very beautiful," says Jane about Donna's entrance into the restaurant.

Though they would soon find themselves romantically involved, their first ever contact was Jane's strong reaction to a comment Donna made about animals.

Donna explains, "Somebody asked me if I did any snorkeling while I was in Turks and Caicos, and I sort of half-jokingly said, 'I did not. I have an irrational fear of wild animals.'"

Jane quickly responded to Donna, raising her voice: "What constitutes a wild animal?"

Donna joshed again, "I don't know, a squirrel?"

"How many squirrels have killed humans versus humans have killed squirrels?" retorted Jane.

Though they clashed for a brief moment at first meeting, the pair quickly made peace and formed a love connection. They now cohabit in southern California.

Jane's strong commitment to the animals, which became clear soon after they met, inspired Donna to explore veganism. Donna says, "When I started dating Jane, and I started seeing her passion for animal rights and veganism, I started to research the subject matter myself." Jane didn't pressure her to become vegan, but by being her bold vegan self, her new partner became curious to learn more. Says Donna, "I just started researching it because I had never been exposed to any of that. I had no idea what was going on with factory farming until I started researching it, and then I understood why she was so passionate and compassionate." Once she learned the truth, Donna went vegan. She explains that watching the short film *Farm to Fridge*, about the cruelty of farming animals, was a turning point for her. "I could never go back to eating meat or dairy again based on what I saw."

Jane says, "I have never met anybody who converted to veganism as quickly as Donna after being open to the information. She's a natural vegan." She adds, "I've dated people who were exposed to the information. I've stuck it in their face and they still didn't change their habits that much. Maybe modified slightly. So I know there are people who are very resistant . . . Donna wasn't that way. Donna's a very compassionate person by nature . . . So as soon as she got the information, it was almost immediate."

Though Donna was inspired by Jane, she points out that her choice to go vegan was based on her own concern for the animals. "If you're doing it for somebody else, it's not going to stick, most likely. It will stick until that somebody ends. But if you're doing it because you have the same beliefs, and you've seen the truth, then it's much more likely to stick. I can never imagine going back," she says.

Donna was quick to become vegan, but Jane hadn't predicted that would happen when the two began dating. Though Jane appreciates being in a relationship with a fellow vegan, she was open to dating a non-vegan. Jane explains that in the past she had "unsuccessful dates with people who snickered at that issue, and one person even sent me a photograph of herself eating a steak. She thought that was funny and I found that repulsive, and that person had no attraction for me. Compassion is the sexiest quality you can have."

By following who she was truly attracted to, without adhering to rigid rules about whether those she dated were vegan, Jane found Donna, a compassionate person whose loving heart led her to veganism.

Jane sees veganism as indicative of other qualities. "It's a sign of being really kind and really responsible and really intelligent. So to me, being vegan is a very attractive quality. It doesn't mean I'm attracted to all vegans, but I do find it to be a very attractive quality. It's like beauty. It's like when somebody's beautiful; vegan is beautiful."

Though Jane enjoys cohabiting with another vegan, she doesn't think all vegans should exclude omnivores from their dating prospects. "I don't want veganism to be this exclusive club that nobody can get into. I would like to open us up to the rest of the world to make them vegan."

Jane encourages women who are dating to be confident in their veganism. According to Jane, "Vegan is sexy. Vegans are sexier than the general population. Your body is purer, you're cleaner, and I'll tell you, you taste better." She adds, "If somebody doesn't want to date you because you're vegan, you don't want to date them. That's for sure."

Going Straight to the Source
Carolyn Malachi, Grammy-Nominated Musician

Accomplished R&B artist Carolyn Malachi came to veganism when she sought to break a negative pattern she saw emerging in her romantic relationships. "I heard someone say that if you experience the same thing with different people, the issue isn't the other people, the issue might be within yourself," she says. "I wanted to get at the root of these relationship issues, and I knew that I had to deal directly with myself, and God." So Carolyn decided to "get rid of the middleman in all areas of my life, including my diet." For the golden-voiced singer that meant getting her energy directly from plants. Many people eat animals such as cattle for their protein, but those animals gather their nutrients from plants. As humans, we have the opportunity to go straight to the source.

Touring the world as a musician, Carolyn has found it simple to maintain her plant-based diet wherever she's stayed, eating lots of fruits and vegetables, and packing vegan snack bars to take with her.

When she's at home in Washington, DC, she finds that her dates often want to impress her with their restaurant choices, but that they don't always take her veganism into consideration. "They want to pick the most glamorous spot in DC. I might look over and see a congressman or congresswoman, but there could be absolutely nothing on the menu that I can [eat]," she explains.

She worried that this might be the case on a recent date with someone who took her to a steak house. *I guess I'll starve*, she thought. But when the waiter came to take their order, her date asked him to bring out every dish that the restaurant could make vegan for them. It was "more food than I could have eaten in two days so that was really sweet. It worked out really well," says Carolyn. Even though he didn't pick a vegan restaurant, her date found a way to be chivalrous about Carolyn's plant-based diet.

Carolyn was previously in a relationship with a fellow vegan which she found to be "refreshing," adding that, "It was really nice to have somebody else in the grocery store who looked at all of the ingredients on the back of the packaging." However, she points out that she is no longer with that person. "Just because one is vegan doesn't mean they're your soul mate."

To vegan women who are considering dating omnivores, she advises, "If you choose to expand your horizons and be with someone who's non-vegan, then know that that might make your relationship or your dating experiences more exciting than you expect them to be. Only if you are both coming to the table with an understanding of each other's needs, then your planning will be based on balance, and it won't be a tug-of-war."

She advises vegan women who worry their veganism will deem them high maintenance, "If you feel that you have to apologize for your life choice to the person you're going out on a date with, then you need to cancel the date, because you should be dating someone who respects your decision, and somebody who wants to be part of your life because they want to add to it, not detract from it."

The "Perfect Vegan" Isn't Always the "Perfect Partner"
Marisa Miller Wolfson, Vegan Activist and Filmmaker

Writer, director, and editor of the award-winning film *Vegucated*, which follows three omnivores as they try a vegan diet, Marisa is directly responsible for inspiring viewers around the world to stop consuming animal products.

Just as Marisa's own film inspired many people to go vegan, a movie originally motivated her to stop eating meat. In 2002, Marisa saw the film *We Are All Noah*, which alerted her to various forms of animal exploitation. "I was blown away and walked away vegetarian," says Marisa. Not long after that, she brought a pamphlet all about veganism with her on a flight. She instantly committed to the cruelty-free lifestyle. "I read it on the plane, and before I touched down, I was vegan."

In her own film, *Vegucated*, Marisa presents important and serious information about veganism in an entertaining way so that non-vegans don't feel attacked. Marisa took the same approach in discussing her compassionate lifestyle with omnivorous love interests when she was single. She is sensitive to listeners' feelings when speaking about veganism and never met a person who wouldn't date her because of her cruelty-free lifestyle.

No date ever interrogated or antagonized Marisa about her veganism, though she did experience some insensitivities. She recounts that one person she dated ". . . ate a meatball sandwich in front of me and I was like, *You really don't get it, you really don't get it.*"

Explains Marisa, "I used to see meat as a 'thing' or a 'food.' I don't see it as such since I went vegan. I don't see 'chicken'; I see parts of a chicken.

I don't see 'pork'; I see parts of a pig. I also know the gruesome process of how the animal got to their plate and what kind of life that animal probably led. So when someone I'm with is eating an animal, all of that flashes in my mind."

As a general rule of thumb, when talking to an omnivore (date or otherwise) about veganism, Marisa opts for honesty. She speaks from the "I" perspective. Says Marisa, "I'm never confrontational . . . If they ask me a question, I will answer no-holds-barred . . . I won't sugarcoat it. But I also won't bash them for . . . what they're doing."

A few weeks after becoming vegan, Marisa first laid eyes on her husband-to-be, David, as he spoke at a forum concerning farm animals. However, she began to date someone else who she met at that same conference—a man who was a devoted vegan, like her. That relationship eventually ended, but Marisa continued to cross paths with David, the two developing a close, fun, meaningful friendship. Soon they began dating, with David disclosing to Marisa early on in their relationship that he was not 100 percent vegan. She has now been with David for more than a decade and the couple has two young vegan children.

David, who is heavily involved in the animal protection movement on a volunteer basis, refers to himself as "veganish." He explains, "Veganish means some shellfish and not being perfect in terms of dairy or eggs when non-vegan food is unavailable."

David teaches animal law, animals and public policy, counsels prominent farm animal protection organizations, and co-drafted ballot initiatives to outlaw some of the cruelest farming practices. Marisa admits that she finds it a little confusing, from her perspective, that someone who has done so much good for animals is not 100 percent vegan, but also recognizes that other leading animal rights activists are not perfect vegans either.

Marisa also points out that her presence has influenced David away from animal products: "David says he's way more vegan from being with me than he was before."

He explains, "I disclose my dietary status in my classes, and I believe my (albeit small) lack of perfection and openness about my diet actually draws people into the movement who otherwise might find the path too intimidating." David confirms he has "moved further along the vegan continuum, in large part due to Marisa, but I have learned from candid conversations with people, many who call themselves 'vegan', that many people who care deeply about animal protection are not always 100 percent consistent and feel pressured to hide any human lapses. I also believe that veganism is not a religion that strives for perfectionism, but a day-to-day choice aimed at doing the best to reduce animal suffering." In David's view, the difference between a 100-percent vegan and a 98-percent vegan "is a difference of 2 percent, not a total failure of conviction or empathy or commitment to reduce animal suffering."

At the end of the day, Marisa and David share a passion for protecting animals. The two also have an undeniable love connection, something that was missing in Marisa's previous relationship with a more stringent vegan. She explains that for ethical vegans, veganism is a "core value," and we look for partners who share these values that are important to us. For the most part, she and David share an avoidance of animal products. But there is more than veganism that brings them together; from their common political views to their shared sense of humor, the pair connect deeply on many levels.

Ultimately Marisa feels, "David is not vegan, but he's . . . 98 percent vegan, and that's good enough for me."

Marisa hopes vegan women who are looking for a partner will "give non-vegan guys a chance, but . . . if there's no budging and if they've seen the movies and read the books, and you can't live with that, it's so understandable if you can't be with that person."

Spreading the Love and Compassion
Krysta Vollbrecht, Works for an Animal Welfare Organization

Vegan since 2007, and living in Portland, Oregon, Krysta Vollbrecht's love for animals plays an important role in both her personal and professional lives. Krysta is unyieldingly honest when it comes to animal issues while maintaining a calm about her that invites people in rather than pushing them away. She outright advocates for veganism when dating, but with a heart full of compassion, not resentment or antagonism.

Krysta initially went vegan following her attendance at a humane education workshop and began working for a farm animal advocacy organization the following year. She says, "I loved my dogs and cats, protested against fur and circuses, but never connected the meat on my plate to the suffering of animals." She adds, "In pursuit of living my best self and aligning my values with my actions, I realized I needed to make my food choices plant-based."

Single and looking when we spoke, Krysta doesn't date vegans exclusively, but prospective partners must at least aspire to be vegan. She explains, "It is painful to watch someone casually choose to buy cheese or eggs when I know, extensively, everything that happened to bring that carton of eggs or block of cheese to the grocery store." And why would Krysta want to be in pain when dating? Dating is about looking for love, not suffering. Instead of subjecting herself to a situation in which she would need to repress who she is and her feelings, Krysta is happy dating people who are only vegan already or open to making the shift someday.

Krysta opts to tell those she is interested in about her ethical lifestyle right away. "It's a big part of my life . . . and since dates usually involve food, I let it be known that I eat vegan so he doesn't invite me to dinner at a steak house." The responses generally reflect her kind attitude. She has found people to be accepting and accommodating and never antagonistic. No one has ever decided not to date her because she is vegan.

Working to convince her dates and partners to go vegan has been routine for Krysta. ". . . Of course I tried to convert them!" she says. "I try to convert everyone! I am happier and healthier than ever living on a plant-based diet. Why wouldn't I want that for everyone?"

Krysta's positive attitude tends to invite questions. And when dates ask them, she has the answers. Krysta doesn't see encouraging a vegan lifestyle as trying to change a person but considers it promoting compassionate decisions. She explains, "It's just the choices we make for which sandwich to eat and which shampoo to buy . . . Some people liken it to religion, but I don't see it that way. You don't change who you are; you just order your latte with soy instead of cow's milk."

"Giving an ultimatum never works: 'Go veg or we can't date,'" suggests Krysta. She did have a positive experience accompanying a partner on his own path, though, and shares that: "At one point, my ex-boyfriend was interested in eliminating dairy (the last of the animal products in his diet) but found it hard. So we did a twenty-one-day vegan kickstart together. We cooked meals together at night, read the motivational emails each morning. I shared vegan cheeses, vegan candy bars, etc. It wasn't him catching up to me; it was something we did together and I think that helped."

Krysta explains that, "It's not always that someone is vegan is such an attraction, but the intention of wanting to make compassionate choices and willingness to grow in that way is so beautiful."

Dos and Don'ts For Dating As a Vegan

Dating as a vegan doesn't have to be difficult. In fact, it can be an opportunity to shine a positive light on veganism. When going out on a date, do be an ambassador for the vegan lifestyle and don't perpetuate the stereotype of the "crazy vegan."

Dos	Don'ts
Communicate and act with respect for all beings, including your date. Show as much compassion for your potential partner as you would any other animal.	Verbally attack your non-vegan date for not sharing your lifestyle.
Have fun getting dressed up in your favorite vegan attire so it sends a visual message about the joys of veganism.	Give your date graphic pamphlets as a visual message about the suffering of animals on factory farms.
Be honest about your beliefs and your reasons for having them.	Tell your date they should go vegan because it's the right thing to do.
Explain your ethical diet before your date picks a place to dine, or suggest a fantastic vegan restaurant.	Agree to eat somewhere and then sit through the meal with your arms crossed because there are no vegan options.
Embrace the possibilities of the unexpected.	Assume a dating prospect will reject your vegan lifestyle.
Answer questions about vegan living calmly and kindly, understanding that the information you are passing on may help animals as well as the person sitting in front of you.	Be condescending or antagonistic when answering questions about veganism.
Be prepared to talk about books and films addressing veganism if your date shows interest.	Demand that your date read books and watch films about veganism against their will.
Be open to love where you find it.	Be too rigid with a long list of qualities you are looking for in a partner.
Expect to be respected and feel free to walk away if you're uncomfortable.	Stay on the receiving end of negativity and aggression.
Have fun!	Be too serious.

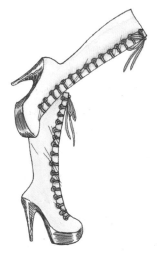

CHAPTER 2

Compassion in Fashion: Dressing Up Without Causing Cruelty

For many women, putting on our favorite outfits and getting ready for dates are exercises in pure fun; when we get dressed, we have the choice of contributing to animal cruelty or wearing our kindness on our sleeves. Veganizing our wardrobes doesn't have to be expensive, and we get to go out into the world knowing that our style didn't come at the expense of an animal's life or well-being.

Kind Clothing

When I went vegan, the changes in my diet came first. Soon after, I took on my closets. I knew that not purchasing any new clothing made with animal products was helping to reduce cruelty, but I really wanted to make a clean sweep. I set out to get rid of any non-vegan products in my home. I wanted to walk around knowing that animals did not suffer for my outfits—including the carefully selected ensembles I wore on dates.

I had basically shopped blindly before I committed to veganism; I paid little attention to what the clothing items I purchased were made from. Once I became conscious of the cruelty, and began to comb through my closets with an awareness of the animal suffering behind certain materials, I was horrified. Just beginning to read the labels of some of my clothes was enough to send shivers down my spine. One fluffy purple scarf had rabbit hairs woven into it. I pictured the bunnies in my mind who suffered for the sake of a scarf. Suddenly what was once a beloved cozy wrap became a scene of violence. After that, it was easy to get rid of.

Piece by piece I reviewed my wardrobe, reading the detailed tags sewn into the seams, or sometimes in the collar, to see what each item was made of. The task felt overwhelming at first but became an act of therapeutic cleansing. Studying the labels on my clothing, and giving away or donating what had been taken from an animal, I began to be connected to the truth and was able to act accordingly. I was no longer unconsciously causing animals pain; I was consciously taking the cruelty out of my closets.

Though I bid some favorite date-wear adieu, I prioritized living a compassionate life and experienced the great reward of knowing my outfits hadn't caused an animal harm.

Getting dressed up can be an important part of going out on a date. Many of us put a great deal of effort into that first visual impression we make when meeting someone we are interested in. And why shouldn't we? Going on a date is an opportunity to show someone our best self, inside and out. We can use clothing as part of how we communicate to others who we are. So don't we want to communicate that we are compassionate people who wouldn't want to hurt other beings?

Since removing the non-vegan clothing from my closets, I have filled them back up with fantastic animal-free clothes. That collection includes many great outfits to wear on dates. And every day, I walk around feeling spiritually lighter knowing that no animal was tortured or killed for what I'm wearing.

When going vegan, many are concerned with the cost of replacing items that are abandoned because they contain animal products. Some people decide to continue wearing non-vegan items until they can afford to replace them. For many, this is a comfortable solution. Others feel that they need to start anew, with a completely vegan wardrobe.

I'll address shoes, coats, and handbags later in this chapter, but for now let's look at veganizing the other elements of your wardrobe. This doesn't have to be an effort that drops your bank account balance to zero.

I've found that it's actually easy to veganize a closet on the cheap, including date-wear. Clothing doesn't have to be expensive. Thrift, resale, consignment, and vintage clothing stores abound, offering reasonable prices with many vegan options. As a nation, we've also turned en masse to what are known as "fast fashion" stores such as Forever 21, Zara, and H&M to fill up our closets while spending very little money. It's true that one could easily veganize their wardrobe on a budget using these stores. They are filled with clothes made from synthetic textiles, with prices often under twenty or even ten dollars. Elizabeth Cline's book *Overdressed* takes a close look at the fast fashion industry and how its incredibly low prices have led to Americans purchasing roughly twenty billion garments per year. The author explains that, without doubt, "to make cheap clothes, you need cheap labor." This has meant that most workers producing these stylish steals have been subjected to less than livable wages and often poor working conditions.

By bypassing the fast fashion stores, we dramatically reduce our negative impact on other people. In buying used clothing instead, we are opting out of a system that sees workers treated unfairly, we are recycling instead of creating more excess, and we are saving money.

The benefits of shopping at used clothing stores are many. They offer the opportunity to purchase new-to-you designer items at a fraction of the original cost. You may also help individuals living with AIDS, homeless animals, women in domestic abuse shelters, and many others in need when shopping at thrift stores that benefit various nonprofit organizations. At used clothing stores, shoppers usually select from clothing that other people have already picked out as desirable: owners and staff at most small secondhand boutiques hand-select what they put on the racks. And remember, the used clothing at those stores once hung in someone else's closet, so that person picked it out too.

A subset of used or secondhand clothing is vintage. Vintage clothing is considered anything that originated in an era prior to the current one. Things like 1940s knee-length skirts, 1970s bell-bottoms, even 1990s plaid flannel shirts are all deemed vintage.

For many, shopping vintage is not a compromise to save money, but a preference. For Alexandra Jacobs, an editor at the *New York Times* who has covered fashion extensively, vintage has been a passion, having held her interest since high school. "I prefer vintage 100 percent for everything but jeans and underwear," she says, explaining that for her vintage is more desirable than new clothes. "I think that what's exciting about vintage is that when you buy a garment, you're not just buying a piece of clothing, you're buying the story behind it . . . If you get something that has been worn before, it's a great way of connecting to the past. There's something very humanizing about it."

Alexandra explains that the quality of vintage is generally superior to fast fashion: "Things are now outsourced and mass produced much more, so these days when we buy something from Old Navy or H&M . . . it's going to fall apart pretty quickly." During the eras when most vintage was produced, "there was much more local production, there was unionization, and the scale was less and so the quality of the material and workmanship tends to be better. Also, people didn't used to shop all the time; people used to shop seasonally. So clothes then were made to last."

All a vegan need do when considering purchasing a used item in person, whether it is vintage or a current style, is read the tag inside the piece of clothing to find out if it contains animal products. This tag is usually found sewn into one of the two main seams inside a piece of clothing and can be located by running your hands along them. If it's not there, it's often sewn into the interior of the collar. Sometimes an item is handmade and lacks a tag, or the information is simply missing. If this is the case, it's up to you to make a judgment call on whether you want to risk taking home an item that might contain an animal product. Recently, I was at a lovely thrift shop in Beacon, New York. I found a gorgeous sleek black Emanuel Ungaro (French designer) dress, in my size, for less than one hundred dollars. I searched along every seam, and around the collar, but could not find out what it was made of. Since this was an elegant evening dress, assembled out of a light and flowing fabric, there was a good chance it was made of silk (not vegan). I put the dress down and walked away from the rack.

Secondhand clothing may also be purchased online, from websites such as Etsy (a collection of independent shops), auction site Ebay, or high-end online resellers such as Vestiaire Collective. When shopping on the Internet, the materials used in a piece of clothing are usually listed. If an item isn't marked vegan, you can contact the seller to confirm whether it contains any animal products.

Shoppers in most secondhand stores do not dig through a random assortment of tossed-away clothing, but rather a carefully curated collection. Like the Dadaists with their readymades, used clothing stores present us with old items in a new light. Saving money, avoiding harm to working people, and the opportunity to unearth designer and vintage gems—who wouldn't want to buy secondhand clothes?

I recently went on a date with my boyfriend to Farm Sanctuary's gala, a fund-raising celebration for the nonprofit organization, and took the opportunity to get as dressed up as possible. My first thought was to purchase a new gown, vegan of course, by a designer whose work I'd coveted for years. In my head I'd made the commitment to indulge in that imagined high-end dress and began to peruse the designer's offerings online. In the meantime, my boyfriend and I took a trip to Miami. After a shopping spree at Melissa, maker of beautiful vegan shoes, we went in search of C. Madeleine, a vintage shop I'd read was like a "museum dedicated to fashion."

When we walked into the store, we were overwhelmed by the massive space housing racks and racks of clothing. It seemed nearly impossible that a building so large could be completely filled with high-quality used clothes.

After picking through the Puccis and settling on a sparkly skirt, I wandered to a back area where my partner was trying on 1970s tuxedo shirts. I looked at the nearby gowns while he was in the dressing room. Suddenly my fingers stumbled across something that caught my attention: a long black dress with rhinestones across the bottom and a magnificent crepe cape on top. A small tag on the inside let me know that it was 100 percent rayon (vegan), so I decided to try it on. Standing in front of the mirror, I felt regal. It was dramatic, glamorous, and unique. And it was from the 1980s (a decade that produced most of my favorite music and fashion). The dress was not cheap, but the price was a quarter of what I would pay for the new gown I had fantasized about.

This was not a dress that a fashion expert conducting a makeover probably would have put me in. It didn't accentuate my waist or perfectly frame my bosom. It wasn't of the moment; in fact, it was thirty years old. But I loved it, and when I came out of the dressing room and let my boyfriend see, he loved it too.

I quickly tossed out the idea of the new designer dream dress and bought my outrageous 1980s glamour gown on the spot.

Some media, parents, and even well-meaning friends will let us think that we need to conform to fashion norms to look good and attract a partner. But in my relationship, I have found that just as it is important to express my true self in regards to veganism, it is important to be myself in respect to fashion. I have discovered that when I buy the clothing that I truly love, the right person for me appreciates my style.

I don't own only used clothing. I still purchase new vegan pieces selectively. There is a lot of great new vegan clothing to be found on the racks of boutiques and online. However, to veganize a wardrobe on a tight budget, used clothing offers great options.

The Cruelty in Our Closets

Being vegan means cutting cruelty to animals out of our lives, wherever it is. That includes our closets. Wool, silk, leather, cashmere, and fur all come from animals. Some wonder if animals must suffer in the production of materials such as wool and silk. For me, there is one clear solution to the question of whether animal-derived clothing is ever ethical: if I refrain from purchasing items made from animal products, I'll be certain that no animal cruelty was involved in their production.

Angora

It is easy to conclude that animals need not suffer when their demise is not a requirement for collecting a textile fiber. Angora is a powerful example of the intense suffering animals endure so that people can take something from them, without causing their death. If you stroke an angora sweater in a store, it will feel soft and inviting, but the reality is that a rabbit was subjected to extraordinary cruelty for it to be made.

When we see the word *angora* on a tag in a piece of clothing, it is referring to the hairs of angora rabbits. People for the Ethical Treatment of Animals (PETA) produced a video that revealed footage of the process sometimes used to collect that hair; rabbits forcibly held, shrieking loudly as their hairs are ripped out by hand. When rabbits are sheared using a tool, they also experience extreme terror and pain, as they are held against their will and often hurt during the process. Regardless of how the hair is removed, the rabbits are kept in captivity, usually suffering with little space to move around, and without proper care.

Can angora hair be collected humanely? Some believe it can. But are we entitled as people to take what belongs to another being for ourselves, without their consent? Will any rabbit be happy held in close quarters, as they generally are on farms?

Walking into a store and picking up an angora sweater, will you know how the rabbits were treated? Can they tell you if they were happy to give up their hair for you to have a sweater? And if a sweater bears a tag claiming that it was ethically made, how will you know what the manufacturer's standards are?

Wool

Most people who encounter sheep at farm animal sanctuaries can tell you they are complex creatures with individual personalities and close relationships with friends and family. Some sheep may not want too much human contact, while others may gently head butt visitors to get more attention. Sheep who live on farm animal sanctuaries are shorn, for their comfort, so many wonder why this wool can't be used to make clothing. Is wearing wool clothing vegan or not?

Just as with angora, or any other animal-derived material, I don't wear wool to ensure that I am not putting on an animal's pain. Though sheep are shorn at sanctuaries for their health and comfort, the industry of raising sheep for wool is flawed and creates great suffering for these sensitive animals.

In the *Animals of Farm Sanctuary* blog, the organization's national shelter director Susie Coston explains, "In the wild, sheep naturally shed their wool and do not require the intervention of humans to shear them." She goes on to elaborate on why sheep bred for wool are shorn: "Those who were domesticated long ago . . . were selectively bred through the years by humans seeking higher wool yields. Sadly, the resultant excess skin and wool only benefits producers who profit at the great expense of sheep."

The only reason the sheep at sanctuaries are shorn is because they have been manipulated by humans to grow an excess of wool. If we continue to support the wool industry, even small farms, sheep will continue to be bred to have unhealthy amounts of wool. The excesses cause myriad health problems including wrinkles that collect urine and serve as a fertile environment for flies to lay eggs—which may cause the potentially deadly condition "fly strike."

To avoid fly strike, many farmers cut off areas of the sheep's skin without anesthetic, a procedure called mulesing. Sheep also endure cuts and terrible emotional distress during the shearing process. According to PETA, "Strips of skin—and even teats, tails, and ears—are often cut or ripped during shearing." This would be a terrifying experience for any animal. For anyone who has experienced the nature of sheep, it is hard to imagine such a gentle being enduring this extreme trauma.

Instead of being part of the cycle of pain, we can be part of the growing momentum toward peace. Giving up a scratchy cable knit sweater is a small price to pay to let an animal live a healthy, happy life. And I have found many bulky, comfy winter sweaters made out of plant-based and synthetic fibers to replace the ones I forfeited when I went vegan.

Silk

The other day I was in a thrift shop trying to find the tag on a piece of clothing I suspected might contain silk. A woman who worked in the store offered to help me. When I explained that I was vegan and didn't wear silk, she asked me what wasn't vegan about silk.

In order to produce silk, the cocoon a silkworm has carefully crafted and is housed in, is treated with hot air, steam, or boiling water, killing the developing insect inside. The protective encasement is then unwound. It is estimated that thousands of silkworms die for every pound of silk produced. Do you really want to wear a piece of clothing created at the expense of so many lives?

When we say no to this cruel fabric, we help reduce the demand. That is a very little way to do a lot of good.

Leather

Leather is made from a number of different animals, including cattle, pigs, sheep, and goats, however, the majority comes from cattle. Some people invest in the idea that leather is simply a by-product of the meat industry and believe that they are putting to use the skins of animals who would have died anyway. The truth is that the leather industry helps keep the meat industry in business, being largely responsible for what makes it profitable. Purchasing leather supports the cruel business of farming these animals for food, which sees millions of them subjected to egregious cruelty such as overcrowding, dehorning, and tail docking before they suffer a frightening and premature death.

Styles of leather include suede, nubuck, patent leather, and chamois. Clothes with any of these descriptive terms on the label contain leather.

There are many leather alternatives available that see no animal suffering. Vegan imitation leather jackets, shoes, handbags, and belts are plentiful at numerous online and brick-and-mortar stores, and they are now frequently made from innovative materials such as cork and pineapple rind. I'll provide more information about purchasing vegan shoes and handbags later in this chapter.

Cashmere

Many associate the word *cashmere* with expensive, luxurious sweaters. These soft fibers are the shorn hair from the underbellies of goats. Though a cashmere sweater may be cozy, it is the result of suffering and pain.

Shearing the goats' underbellies denies them their natural protection and leaves them exposed to the cold. According to HappyCow.net,

"Typically, the goats are raised in filthy, crowded conditions, ear notched, dehorned, and castrated without anesthesia." As many as 50 to 80 percent of goats farmed for cashmere are killed at a young age because their coats are deemed "defective." That doesn't sound too cozy, does it?

Shearling

There is nothing cruelty-free about shearling. Just one of these coveted coats can require the hides of dozens of sheep. Though some believe shearling is made from sheared wool (also not cruelty-free), it is actually the skin of slaughtered sheep with the wool still on it. Sliding on a shearling jacket may make one feel impervious to the cold, but in fact those who wear them are wrapping themselves in the suffering of others.

Fur

It's hard to find a person these days who isn't aware of the cruelties of fur. But many still wear it, and the industry is still going strong, even with so many beautiful, high-quality fake furs available.

Animals who are slaughtered for their fur are killed in incredibly cruel ways including suffocation, gas, and poison, as well as anal and vaginal electrocution. On fur farms, they endure terrible living conditions before experiencing a particularly traumatic death. The suffering is the same whether their fur is used for the pompom on a winter hat or collects thousands of dollars as part of a full-length coat.

Some animals killed for their fur are trapped in the wild. In these cases, they often live through intensely painful and terrifying conditions including (but not limited to) dehydration, blood loss, shock, and attacks by predators before finally losing their lives.

Despite the amount of cruelty involved, many people still flaunt their fur. But the more of us who keep it out of our closets, the less suffering the industry will cause.

Down

A lot of children have "blankies"—small blankets that they demand be present if they are going to take a nap or settle down to sleep.

I didn't have a blankie; I had a "feather pillow." What I now know was a down pillow, created with cruelty, was my inanimate sleep-time companion. I had no idea that my comfort was coming at the cost of someone else's pain.

When I took on a compassionate lifestyle, it took me a moment to figure out that my beloved down items were not vegan and were cruelly produced. Down is actually a layer of feathers on birds, close to their skin. I relied on down for winter coats (as well as my feather pillows), not realizing that my warmth was the result of the suffering of ducks and geese. To collect down, these elegant and sentient beings are often held in crowded, dirty conditions and plucked alive. Far from a painless process, the frightened birds are left with significant wounds.

Although some claim to produce down items that are cruelty-free, made with the feathers that have naturally fallen off of birds, it is hard to believe that the down industry can be sustained without ducks and geese suffering. With the amount of down consumed internationally, I can't envision a world where all of those blankets and jackets have been produced by the feathers that have naturally fallen off of birds.

There are many warm alternatives to down, and no reason a duck or a goose, who would be much happier splashing in a lake, should have to live in crowded conditions enduring live-plucking for a winter coat or a feather pillow.

Shoes, Handbags, and Coats

When I went vegan, I lugged bags full of leather and suede shoes to my best friend's house, letting her have whatever she wanted. Everything leftover I gave to a local thrift shop. I knew I couldn't afford to replace all of the shoes right away, but I wanted them out of my house. I wanted to reduce the animal cruelty in my home as much as possible.

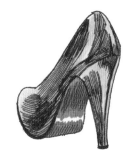

What to do with leather shoes and handbags is a difficult question for many women who go vegan. We want to be "good vegans," but we don't want to leave ourselves without a nice selection of accessories. Shoes and purses can be expensive, and those of us without large incomes may not be able to purchase the replacements we want without saving money for some time.

For some, the expense of buying new shoes and handbags means we hold on to our old leather items until we can afford vegan versions. This way we don't support cruelty and can veganize our wardrobe in a stress-free manner when funds are sufficient. For others, we cannot bear to house the cruelly produced products in our homes, and we prioritize purchasing vegan replacements as soon as possible.

Shoes

There are some wonderful sources for vegan footwear. MooShoes, a cruelty-free shoe store with locations in New York City and Los Angeles, is a favorite among many vegans (they ship internationally). However, if you don't have access to a vegan shop, or are looking for alternatives, animal-free shoes can be found in plenty of non-vegan shoe stores.

For a while after committing to a compassionate lifestyle, I limited myself to vegan shoe stores. Then one day, a vegan friend mentioned something over coffee that changed my shoe-shopping outlook. She told me she had just been at the major shoe store chain DSW. "They have vegan shoes at DSW?" I asked. "Yes," she explained, "if you can read small labels and have an hour or so to find them."

That's when I discovered that most shoes bear a stamp indicating what they are made of. The information about what materials have been used is often inside the shoe and easy to read. If the stamp indicates that the whole shoe is composed of "man-made" materials, they should not contain leather.

Shopping online, one can usually find out what shoes are made of in their description. Another very important tool for vegans is the label on many shoes composed of little pictures. This is a great key to whether the shoes contain animal products. If you don't see the label immediately, check the inside or the sole of the shoe. If it isn't there, look at the shoebox. It could also be there.

The label will have images on it that look something like those in the illustration below:

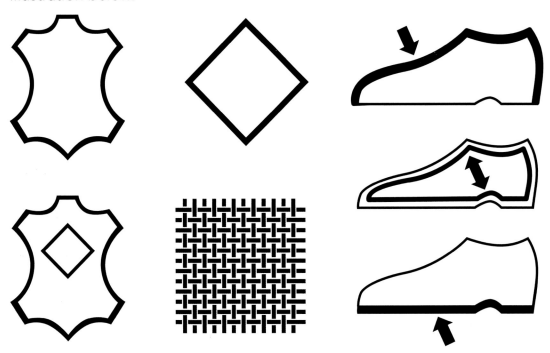

The three images on the right describe different parts of the shoe. The first image is the "upper." The second image is the "lining and sock," and the third image is the "outer sole."

To the left of those images, more importantly, are the images that tell us what the shoe is made of. We see the symbol for "leather" in the upper left, the image for "coated leather" is below it, the image for "textile" is in the middle bottom, and the image for "other materials" is in the center on top.

footwear

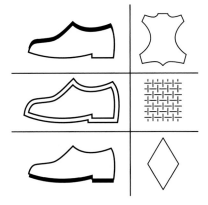

To the right is a sample label that uses this system:

From this label, you can see that the upper is made of leather, the lining and sock are made of textile, and the outer sole is made of other materials. Since it contains leather, this shoe is definitely not vegan.

Now, the label or stamp doesn't tell us if any animal products have been used in the glue or any other elements of the shoe (such as the laces). So when using this system, we need to use our own judgment to decide if a shoe fits our vegan standards.

Of course if you shop at a vegan store, you can be sure that all of the shoes are free of animal products. MooShoes is still my favorite source for vegan footwear, but it's nice to know that I have options. In addition to DSW, some non-vegan stores that have plenty of vegan shoes are Steve Madden (I have had the most luck with their Madden Girl collection), the Zappos website (try searching "vegan"), and Nine West. Another little known source for vegan footwear is the Etsy website. There are many enticing offerings from independent sellers if you simply search "vegan shoes" on this abundant site, which is focused on hand-crafted and vintage items. Etsy can be a great option if you are on a budget, as the vintage vegan shoes tend to be affordable, usually priced between twenty and fifty dollars.

Handbags

I love handbags and purses. I have a number of them; however, I tend to use the same ones over and over. Handbags are fun accessories, but we don't require many of them to get through life (though we may want a lot of them). In removing the non-vegan handbags from my wardrobe, I was only left with a few purses. But that was enough for me to get by until I could afford to buy new ones.

Though brand-new, high-quality vegan handbags can run into the hundreds of dollars (or cost more than $1,000 if Stella McCartney is your designer of choice), there are some great options for less expensive bags. As with clothing, shopping secondhand can be a great way to find affordable, high-quality vegan handbags while avoiding fast fashion.

Just last week I purchased a gorgeous red, marbleized Lucite evening purse at my favorite used clothing store, Vintage: Beacon, for $69.50. If that sounds like a little too much, I also found an adorable black fabric purse with a raised pattern at Housing Works (a thirft shop) in New York City for $15. The eBay website is a wonderful resource for used cruelty-free handbags. Type "Matt & Nat" (a brand of beautiful vegan purses) in the search field to find a great selection of used bags often priced at $20 or less. You may also want to get creative with your searches. Try searching "Lucite purse" and see what you find, or "straw purse." Remember that once you've left the realm of vegan brands, you'll need to read the details or contact the seller to find out if a purse is completely vegan.

Coats

Coats were a conundrum for me when I first went vegan. I lived in New York City, with brutally cold winters, and had owned down coats for as long as I could remember. I wasn't quite sure what I was going to do to get through winters without wearing animal products.

Enter Vaute. I was so pleased to discover the company that Leanne Mai-ly Hilgart founded in 2008. She is the maker of a whole line of beautiful, warm, ethically made, vegan winter coats. Leanne is from the Chicago area so she has a great deal of experience with frigid winters. Her coats protect me from even the fierceness of an upstate New York February.

A Vaute coat is worth every penny in my experience, but may not be in everyone's price range. There are other options for those of us on a tight budget. I found my first vegan coat at Burlington Coat Factory when I was subsisting on a relatively slight income. I went through the racks, reading the tags on coats that were within my price range, until I found a vegan one that I liked. Yes, it required some extra effort, but it was a small price to pay to walk out knowing I hadn't paid into the suffering of animals.

When seeking out a vegan coat, be sure to stay aware of trims. Fur collars have a way of sneaking in, even on otherwise cruelty-free coats. And those trims are a lot of cruelty on a little bit of coat.

Putting On Our Vegan Best

When I was in my thirties, I took a job as a publicist and had the pleasure of working on world-renowned fashion expert Tim Gunn's book *Tim Gunn: A Guide to Quality, Taste & Style*. Of course I read it cover to cover. The book provided detailed directions for cleaning out a closet. During my leave from the job due to cancer, I followed those instructions step by step, with my mother's help. Amazingly, the contents of my closet decreased by about 60 percent. I was no longer fighting my way through stuffed-together dresses and items I hadn't worn in years sticking out in every direction.

A simple philosophy presented by Gunn turned my closet from an overwhelming mess to a more manageable and inviting collection. What I learned from the book was to only keep what made my heart sing, with very few exceptions. Gunn advises to do "no agonizing over whether or not to keep the jumpsuit. If you have to ask, the answer is: Throw it away." In the closet-cleaning process, he advises readers to hold on to those items that create "heart palpitations of happiness . . ." When I let go of almost everything else, I ended up with a wardrobe I loved. In a shop, trying on clothing, there will often be a piece that causes me to tilt my head from side to side, trying to figure out if I want it. Now I know *that* is a good sign to put the dress back on the rack. Individuals in America buy an average of sixty-four items of clothing a year. Why do we need all of those clothes? We are simply creating more waste. If we buy only what we love, we will cut down considerably.

In an article published by *The Atlantic* website, *Overdressed* author Cline shares, "Americans send 10.5 million tons of clothing to landfills every year." This isn't because no one is purchasing the clothing from secondhand shops; it is because it isn't getting to them in the first place. According to the same article by Cline, "Americans recycle or donate only 15 percent of their used clothing." The rest goes in the garbage. If we reduce what we buy, and donate what we don't want anymore, we will not only make our own lives easier, but we will also help save the planet.

I find that when I follow Gunn's advice to keep only what I love, getting dressed for dates is a whole lot easier. I don't open my closet to an overwhelming wall of clothing, but rather to a carefully selected assortment of pieces that make me happy. Who wants to meet someone we're excited about while wearing something that makes us feel mediocre?

My philosophy when it comes to dressing for dates is to not negate who I am, but to put the best version of myself forward. For me, it's not about looking "put together" in a generic matter that works for everyone, but putting in an effort and turning up the volume on what I like about me. So I may not wear a black fitted dress with spaghetti straps and sweetheart neckline that would probably make anyone look good, but I may pull out my favorite red dress that I bought at a thrift shop, steam it so that it looks great, and combine it with a chunky necklace. It is an expression of who I am, I feel good in it, and my boyfriend loves that dress.

It gets funny when you start to look around at couples. For years, I bought into the idea that I needed to dress a certain way (as I saw depicted on some television shows, and described by friends) to find a match. But reality proved me wrong. A friend of mine, let's call her Edie, is my personal fashion icon. She has a devoted partner with whom she shares a love of literature, art, and music. And he loves her unique look. I have never once seen her in an outfit that would be featured as the end result of a magazine makeover. She is often in free-flowing dresses that lack waistlines, with costume jewelry and clunky shoes adorning her feet. Dressing in what makes her happy, and not buying into fashion propaganda, Edie had no problem finding a partner who appreciated her and her style.

What we wear can be an important means of self-expression. Just as with veganism, if we hide who we really are, we may miss out on meeting someone who appreciates our true selves.

Just look at the hugely successful comedian Tig Notaro. I've never once seen her photographed or filmed in a dress or skirt. Pants and a shirt (sometimes with a jacket) seem to be her uniform. I am going to guess that if she were subjected to popular makeover standards, she would be made unrecognizable. But who wants Tig to be unrecognizable? She is a cancer survivor, an accomplished performer, and an incredible role model for women everywhere. Why can't she wear pants and a shirt on a date? I have a feeling that her date would prefer Tig dress as she wants.

In fashion, just as with veganism, I have found what works best for me is to be honest with others about who I am. I pay attention to my feelings when I'm getting dressed, and I know if my outfit is making my heart sing or if I feel uncomfortable.

Media makeovers aren't all bad, though, when approached mindfully. Danielle Legg, who we'll get to know better in chapter 4, has a lot to say about television makeovers. She was the subject of one that aired on the nationally syndicated program *Dr. Phil*.

In her late twenties, a single and looking Danielle appeared in a *Dr. Phil* segment, receiving dating advice and a makeover from Patti Stanger, star of television show *The Millionaire Matchmaker*. Stanger suggested that Danielle dress up more for dates. Danielle thought that if she had to dress up to attract someone, maybe she didn't want to be with that person. However, she felt great in her makeover outfit and decided to take some of the pointers to heart. "Initially I took that advice—and it did change the way I dressed. After the show, the man that was my best friend ended up asking me on a few dates. I dressed the hell outta those dates. I wore dresses and heels, I wore makeup! Prior to the show I didn't wear dresses at all, ever . . . I learned that without the perfect body, I could feel great about myself when I wore a dress," she says. Though Danielle discovered dresses as a result of the makeover, she wore them because they made her feel good. Eventually she found a balance between the makeover look and what she felt portrayed her authentic self. She says, "For every date, I give that person a realistic, honest look at me, from everything on the inside to the outermost layer of my clothing." Though she continues to wear some dresses, Danielle has traded in the heels for Converse sneakers.

The makeover wasn't a terrible experience for Danielle, and she did take away some useful tips, but when dressing for dates, her personal style choices reign. Though Danielle took the advice to turn up the volume on her true beauty, she did it in an honest way, not donning outfits that denied her real nature, but providing a portrait of her best self.

Danielle says, "If I'm wearing something I don't like, or that I'm not comfortable in, it changes the whole dynamic of me—I'm too busy in my head thinking about my clothes to enjoy myself. I have to be true to me . . ."

Fashion tips from media and people we know can deny us our true selves or highlight them. But if we listen to our hearts, and stick with what we love, we won't be wearing a lie, but an expression of who we are.

When I found a partner who appreciated me, I discovered that he enjoyed my personal style, too. He doesn't always love what I wear, but more often than not we agree on my favorite outfits.

I'm not saying that we can't potentially distance ourselves from people by wearing clothing that could make them feel uncomfortable, though. A first date may not be the ideal moment to wear our most outrageous pieces of clothing. However, if that outfit is what truly makes you happy then perhaps you want a significant other who will embrace it as much as you do. Clothing definitely has the power to alienate others or draw them near. Most of the time, if we take a moment to listen to our feelings, we can tell when we look in the mirror if something we're wearing might push someone away. If we make an effort to be true to ourselves, we will be more likely to attract people who like us for who we are and reflect those qualities. The clothing that speaks to you will probably speak to someone else, too.

Quick Guide: Vegan/Not Vegan Materials

For those who feel that going vegan will deprive you of incredible, beautifully made clothing, fear not! Fantastic vegan fabrics abound. What follows are lists of materials that are vegan-friendly, and those that are not. You can bring this along with you when you go shopping.

Vegan	Not Vegan
Acrylic	Angora
Bamboo	Cashmere
Cotton	Fur
Hemp	Leather (including suede, nubuck,
Jute	patent leather, chamois, calfskin)
Linen	Shearling
Modal	Silk
Nylon	Snake, lizard, and other skins
Polyester	Wool
Ramie	
Rayon	
Spandex	

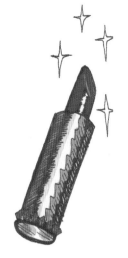

CHAPTER 3

De-Bugging Your Beauty Routine: Vegan Makeup

Not all women wear makeup, but for those of us who do, we often devote a lot of time and energy to putting it on, especially when we're going on a date. I usually begin to plan what cosmetics I'm going to wear when I pick out an outfit for a special occasion. For many of us, it is a fun and important part of preparing for a big night out with a partner or meeting someone new.

Although many cosmetics contain animal products, or were tested on animals, there is an abundance of cruelty-free and vegan makeup available. There's no need to worry—with an all-vegan makeup collection, as Prince said, "U Got the Look."

Vegan Visage

I committed to a vegan lifestyle in February 2008. My dietary changes were immediate. I had been vegetarian for the year prior, and the moment I made the decision to go completely cruelty-free, I stopped eating eggs, consuming dairy, or opting for any other animal products in my food.

Once my eyes opened to the cruelty in my lifestyle, the food came first. The clothing was soon to follow. But I knew that animal suffering was not limited to what I ate and wore. My bathroom contained a cornucopia of cosmetics. I loved the whole process of putting on makeup, from the inception of the look, to digging through my collection, to brushing on the colors. Sometimes I applied a natural look, other times I painted on more dramatic shades. When I was in my twenties, I liked to put on blue eyeshadow with tiny gold stars glued on top—my version of a starry night. I didn't realize that the glue I used was likely the result of animal suffering.

The people I've been in relationships with have also appreciated my face paint. One person I dated in college remarked that I always had a little bit of glitter somewhere. It may have been true at the time, as I often enjoyed a bit of sparkle.

When I went vegan, I was surprised to discover that most of these products are built on cruelty. Their crimes against animals are two-fold. Many cosmetics companies test their products on guinea pigs, mice, rabbits, hamsters, and rats, causing them excruciating pain and death.

Makeup that hasn't been tested on animals still often contains products derived from them. Some common ingredients often found in makeup include carmine (the result of crushing cochineal insects), beeswax (harvested from the honeycombs of bees), and guanine (derived from fish scales).

Today, most brands that are vegan-friendly (selling some vegan products) publish information about their animal-free offerings on the Internet, but at the time of my shift to a cruelty-free lifestyle, those details were not so freely available. So a few weeks after going vegan, I dumped my makeup collection onto my bed and organized the little containers by brand. Then I emailed each company to find out whether those seemingly innocent eye shadows, lipsticks, blushes, eyeliners, mascaras, and foundations were in fact vegan.

As the responses arrived, I found myself relieved. Though the process meant forsaking some of my favorite shades, I would no longer be putting on a cruel face. Who wants to walk around with crushed bugs highlighting her cheeks anyway? Not me. No gold glittering shadow was worth the suffering of a bunny rabbit.

When I looked at my makeup collection, spread out on a towel on my bed, the task of contacting each cosmetics company seemed daunting. But as I went through the steps to research what was and wasn't vegan, I felt eager to find out the truth. I was excited to cut the cruelty out of my cosmetics collection.

Most of the companies I contacted responded to my inquiries, and I threw out any product that wasn't vegan or I was uncertain about. Once the job was complete, I felt great about my all-vegan collection. Moving forward, I researched whether makeup was vegan before purchasing it. Now I usually buy from brands that make the information easily accessible.

When I first went vegan, with a little research, I found some companies that were as committed to a vegan lifestyle as I was and some that offered vegan options. When I cleared the cruelty from my collection, I found plenty of vegan products with which to replenish my makeup bag. I purchased numerous items from Arbonne, Ecco Bella, Beauty Without Cruelty, and Urban Decay. Today, there are even more vegan and vegan-friendly brands, offering products ranging from natural-looking blushes, to gloriously glam lipsticks, to perfectly punk-rock eye shadows.

Now my makeup cup runneth over. I have eye shadows in shades ranging from sparkly beige to deep turquoise, and lipsticks in pinks, reds, purples, and browns. I do not want for anything that's not vegan, because so much available is animal-free.

Just as with food, and with my clothing, when I followed what I knew to be right in my heart, continuing to clear the cruelty from my makeup collection despite challenges, I ended up with wonderful vegan options.

I still love wearing makeup and my current boyfriend appreciates my vegan visage. His adoration is not my main motivation for putting on cosmetics, but I do enjoy the compliments.

U Got the Look: A Classic Face by Makeup Master Brian Duprey

Brian Duprey has been a professional makeup artist for twenty-six years, and vegan for thirty. His steady hand has helped models look stunning in magazines including *Vogue*, *Elle*, *Marie Claire*, and *W*.

In addition to mastering the art of makeup application, Brian is an authority on vegan products. He offers his favorite professional vegan and cruelty-free makeup tips for achieving a stunning overall look.

Brian's Suggested Products:

Eye shadow
Brand: Pacifica
Product: Super Powder Supernatural Eye Shadow Trio
Shade: Stone, Cold, Fox

Brand: Pacifica
Product: Enlighten Eye Brightening Shadow Palette

Brand: Juice Beauty
Product: Phyto-Pigments Cream Shadow Stick
Shade: Cove

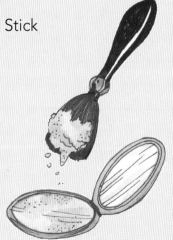

Blush
Brand: The All Natural Face
Product: Cream Blush
Shade: Match to your complexion

Brand: E.L.F.
Product: Powder Blush Palettes
Shade: Match to your complexion

Concealer
Brand: Tarte
Product: Maracuja Creaseless Concealer
Shade: Match to your complexion

Foundation
Brand: Nars
Product: Sheer Glow Foundation
Shade: Match to your complexion

Loose Powder
Brand: Urban Decay
Product: Naked Skin Ultra Definition Loose Finishing Powder
Shade: Match to your complexion

Mascara
Brand: Tarte
Product: Lights, Camera, Lashes 4-in-1 Mascara

Lip color
Brand: Obsessive Compulsive Cosmetics
Product: Lip Tar
Shade: Pick a shade that complements, not overpowers

Brushes
Brand: Ecotools

Tips From Brian:

Prep
Shape eyebrows.
Use an eyelash curler to curl lashes.

Complexion

Dab concealer onto brush. Brush and pat into needed areas. These are generally under the eye, around nostrils, and any discolored spots.

If the foundation does not have an attached applicator, use a foundation brush to apply for a smooth, sheer finish. Brush over entire face, spreading out a small amount, and applying over eyelids and brow bone. Apply with brushstrokes where less coverage is necessary and pat brush to build more coverage where needed.

With your finger or a foundation brush, apply cream blush to the apple of your cheek and blend out. I use my foundation brush that still has a little foundation on it to blend cream blush.

Pat small amount of loose powder over the face. I use Powder Puffs from Alcone Pro store that can be tossed in the wash. Remember, a glow on the cheek adds life to the complexion, so don't over-powder.

Eyes

Apply Juice Beauty Phyto-Pigments Cream Shadow Stick directly to eyelid or use a medium eye shadow brush, blending the cream shadow over your lid and through the crease, then up toward brow until seamless. Once done, pat a small amount of loose powder on eyelid to absorb the oils in the product.

With a different eye shadow brush, apply your favorite powder eye shadow in the same placement as the cream shadow. Layering these products will give you a longer wear and better eye shadow payoff than just using one alone. I love to use Pacifica Super Powder Supernatural Eye Shadow Trio (Stone, Cold, Fox) and Enlighten Eye Brightening Shadow Palette. For a flawless finish, use your foundation brush with a little foundation left on it to brush across brow bone, blending shadow and lightly highlighting the brow bone.

Apply mascara in your preferred amount and comb through with a metal lash comb between coats. I use a waterproof formula on top to lock in the curl.

Use a brow pencil that is a direct match to your hair color. With very little pressure, gently stroke the pencil through your brow and brush through with an eyebrow brush once done.

Blush

If the cream blush is too sheer for you, layer over it with your favorite powder blush. I love E.L.F. Powder Blush Palettes for the multiple shades per palette.

Keep blush sheer—you don't want to matte your cheek when using a powder blush; a glow should still show through.

Lips

Finish your best natural look with any shade of lip tar from Obsessive Compulsive Cosmetics. A little goes a long way and they have every shade under the sun. Choose a color that complements, not over-powers.

Demystifying Makeup

Once I began to research what wasn't vegan about my makeup collection, I discovered that my cosmetics contained a variety of animal products including carmine and beeswax. Products that didn't include these cruel contents might have been tested on innocent animals. Rather than swear off makeup entirely, I dove in and learned more about which products were tested on animals, what were the common animal-derived ingredients, and how I could tell if a product was vegan.

Animal Testing

Unfortunately many cosmetics are tested on animals. Animals used for testing are sub-jected to numerous painful experiments. Some endure substances dripped into their eyes,

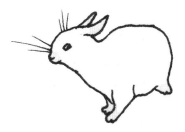

while others are force-fed massive doses of a chemical, among other excruciating procedures. Despite the availability of cruelty-free non-animal tests, Humane Society International (HSI) estimates that every year as many as 100,000 to 200,000 animals are put through these sometimes lethal experiments for the sake of selling cosmetics. HSI reports that even if the process itself doesn't result in death, animals are killed following the test.

As numerous vegan and cruelty-free companies have demonstrated, this painful and deadly testing process is completely unnecessary. Many countries have banned animal testing, further proving that there is no need to subject animals to the tests, yet the practice is still legal in many places.

Common Culprits: Ingredients That Hurt

There are many animal products that may be found in makeup and perfumes. Some cosmetics ingredients may have been sourced from an animal or a plant, such as stearic acid, which could come from either. Though the animal ingredients found in makeup are numerous, a few common culprits frequently appear in products. If you see one of these included on an ingredients list, you'll know immediately that the item is not vegan.

Ambergris—Is your perfume vegan? Not if it contains this ingredient. Ambergris is produced in the intestinal tract of whales and is often used as a fragrance fixative in perfumes. Is any scent worth an animal's suffering?

Beeswax—The name says it all. Beeswax is a secretion of bees and used in products ranging from lipsticks to mascaras. Not only are the bees held in captivity against their will to obtain beeswax, but many have their wings cut, or are killed as part of the process.

Carmine—This red coloring comes from crushed cochineal insects. Many cosmetics companies rely on the use of carmine for pink and red shades. You can opt out of contributing to the death of these innocent insects by choosing companies that use vegan alternatives.

Guanine—Derived from fish scales, Guanine can often be found in lipsticks, nail polishes, and mascaras. Completely unnecessary, many animal-free options abound for creating the perfect vegan face.

Lanolin—Mostly found in makeup we wear on our lips, like lipsticks and glosses, lanolin is a wax secreted by the oil glands of sheep. With the vast array of vegan lip colors available, it is easy to keep lanolin out of your makeup bag.

Musk—The moment I read "musk" on a perfume's ingredients list, my heart sinks. Found in many fragrances, musk is collected from the glandular secretions of animals including musk deer, civet cats, and beavers. The animals from who the musk is collected are frequently killed, though in some cases they live through a painful extraction.

Tallow—Often found in foundations, lipstick, and eye makeup, tallow is the rendered fat of slaughtered animals. That is quite a high price to pay for a made-up face. Why wear someone's pain when there are so many animal-free options?

The best way to ensure that makeup is vegan is to stick with cosmetics labeled as such, or with companies that are all-vegan or vegan-friendly. If your cosmetics case contains a product you purchased previous to going vegan and you are uncertain of its status, you can always email customer service to ask if it contains animal products and whether it was tested on animals. Most of the companies I contacted were quick to reply.

Cruelty-Free and Vegan Makeup

Generally when we use the term *cruelty-free* we think, *vegan*. However, in the world of cosmetics, *cruelty-free* and *vegan* mean two different things.

As applied to cosmetics, the term *cruelty-free* means that a product was not tested on animals. It may still contain animal products such as carmine, lanolin, or beeswax, and therefore not be vegan. Some companies may label their products "cruelty-free," while still using ingredients that have been tested on animals.

Products that are vegan contain no animal products. However, a product that is vegan may still have been tested on animals and therefore not be cruelty-free.

WHAT?

Different cosmetics companies have different standards for labeling their products "cruelty-free," and vegans have varying standards for makeup they will use. Personally, I seek out products that are both cruelty-free (product and ingredients not tested on animals) and vegan (containing no animal products).

You always have the option of contacting a cosmetics company to find out if a particular product is vegan and cruelty-free. However, a few organizations have gone through the trouble of establishing whether products are cruelty-free or vegan for you. If you see one of these logos on a product, you will know that item has already been subject to a rigorous review establishing whether it is cruelty-free or vegan.

The chart on the next page will guide you through some of the labels that appear on makeup. If a different logo is used, it may not represent the high standards of the organizations listed on the chart. These are established groups that have earned the trust of vegans around the globe.

Let's Go Shopping

I love shopping for makeup. The colors, the textures, the idea of looking glamorous, fresh-faced, or slightly shimmery excites me. I enjoy imagining what shadow I might wear to a cocktail party, or which lipstick could go perfectly with a new dress. But walking into a large makeup chain or department store without knowing in advance which items are vegan and cruelty-free can be stressful and frustrating. Without coming prepared, a makeup shopping spree can be a total wash.

I've asked for help from salespeople at large makeup chains and department store cosmetics counters and have been misguided on a number of occasions, purchasing items only to discover later that they are not vegan. If we want our makeup to be cruelty-free and vegan, our best bet is to rely on our own research or purchase makeup that is clearly labeled by a

 Certified Vegan	• No animal-derived ingredients • Products, formulations, and individual ingredients not tested on animals
 Choose Cruelty Free (CCF)	• Products, formulations, and individual ingredients not tested on animals
 Leaping Bunny	• Products, formulations, and individual ingredients not tested on animals
 PETA Cruelty-Free	• Products, formulations, and individual ingredients not tested on animals
 PETA Cruelty-Free and Vegan	• No animal-derived ingredients • Products, formulations, and individual ingredients not tested on animals
 The Vegan Society	• No animal-derived ingredients • Products, formulations, and individual ingredients not tested on animals

U Got the Look: Bold Lips by Cosmetics Innovator Chad Michael Maxwell

Chad Michael Maxwell, a committed vegan, acquired the nickname Color Me Chad during his eleven years as a makeup artist for well-known cosmetics brands. In 2010, he moved (with his now vegan partner) to Brooklyn, New York. Working as a freelance artist for fashion shows, photo shoots, music videos, and television, Chad found himself frequently placed in the position of purchasing products against his vegan ethics. He decided to create what he and many others were seeking: high-quality vegan and cruelty-free lipstick. Using his nickname, he formed Color Me Chad LLC in 2011 and began his amazing journey of making vegan lipstick.

Lipstick Tips From Chad:

Isn't it great that in addition to being conscious of cosmetic ingredients and their sources, we have also moved further away from the structured rigid rules that dictated to us for so long what beauty is allowed to be? A fun example of this is seeing more than just classic red or safe nude lips at red carpet and formal events. We could talk about "rules" for makeup all day (and I wouldn't be saying anything new).

Most people I talk to are still not sure how to pick the "right" red. For reds, find one that matches your complexion (yellow tones for skin with yellow in it, blue tones for skin with more blue in it, etc.) for a more natural look, or the opposite for a bolder look. Don't make it more complicated than that. I believe confidence is how you wear any color.

Confidence starts with great application. So here are my favorite tips for how to get it on right:

Crazy smile

For your first application especially, to avoid skips, make an open-mouthed smile. This holds your lips tight and in place during application, giving you full coverage that should make future touch-ups easier.

Same direction

It doesn't matter if you work from in to out or out to in, just use the same direction for each half of your lips. This will give you the most even application.

Translucent powder

Use translucent powder under any lipstick to create a matte finish and help it last longer. The powder will not change the lipstick color and helps absorb excess oils so it not only stays on longer, but also stays in place.

There's no lipstick police, so don't be afraid to try a new and different color!

trustworthy organization (such as with the logos listed earlier in this chapter). And remember, just because makeup is labeled cruelty-free, doesn't mean that it's vegan.

On a recent summer's day I went on a vegan (no animal ingredients or testing) makeup shopping spree in New York City. My first stop was Sephora, near Manhattan's Union Square. With some simple preparation, I stocked up on numerous delightful vegan goodies at this popular chain shop. Kat Von D is veganizing her entire line of makeup, which can be found at Sephora. I love her vegan Studded Kiss Lipstick and liquid Tattoo Liner for eyes. If you are going to a Sephora in search of Kat Von D makeup, simply visit her website ahead of your trip, and you will find a full list of her vegan products.

At the same store, I found Argan Enlightenment Illuminizer by Josie Maran, a luscious cream that adds a little shimmer to the face or body, perfect to rub (sparingly) all over for a beach date. I found out it was vegan by emailing the company ahead of time to ask which of Maran's products are animal-free. My Sephora bag of goodies also included a gorgeous eye shadow by Nars and colorful lipsticks from Too Faced. Hourglass is another brand found in Sephora stores that is vegan-friendly (offering vegan options). Nars customer service was quick to let me know which products were vegan, while Hourglass and Too Faced both provide information about their vegan items online.

I stepped out into the sunny day and made my way down to the E.L.F. Cosmetics store in the East Village. Though all E.L.F. makeup is vegan, some of their skin care products and brushes are not. Given their massive line of cosmetics, that leaves a lot to choose from. E.L.F. products are very reasonably priced, and I walked out of the store with a bag of more than ten items for less than $50.

Stepping into a Lush shop is like wandering into a not-so-secret garden of enchanting scents. Best known for their bath products, Lush stores smell divine with a delicious perfume that wafts onto the street when one walks past. I entered the welcoming shop to select from their vegan makeup options. Though not everything in the store is vegan, much of it is, and none of it is tested on animals.

After so much shopping, I was tired, but determined to pick up some vegan perfume. I hopped on a subway uptown to the famous Macy's department store. I was in search of popular clothing brand Juicy Couture's line of scents, and I knew I would find it there. I had recently read that all the company's perfumes had been made completely vegan. It sounded too good to be true, so I spoke to a customer service representative. He assured me that they do not test on animals, nor do the perfumes contain any animal products. I was so excited that I asked him twice. He confirmed, both times. At Macy's, I sniffed my way through Juicy Couture's offerings and purchased my favorite, Viva La Juicy.

Health-food stores often carry vegan makeup brands (like ZuZu Luxe) and some that are vegan-friendly (like Ecco Bella). For those of us who do not live near a health-food store or a Sephora, many Target stores (and chain drugstores) offer products by all-vegan brand Pacifica, and from companies with some vegan items like Wet N Wild (which lists vegan products on its website) and E.L.F.

But if there is no Target near you, not a health-food store in sight, and Sephora isn't within driving distance, there is a vast selection of cruelty-free vegan makeup available for purchase on the Internet. Though we can't try on makeup we purchase online before buying it, we can generally get a good idea of what it will look like from photos. One of the benefits of purchasing online is that you can buy from small brands that are not available in big chain retailers. I recently ordered from a number of vegan and vegan-friendly cosmetics companies and was delighted when the packages came in the mail.

Not too long ago, it was challenging to find the perfect pink vegan blush. Many cosmetics companies had relied on non-vegan carmine for the reddish shades of their makeup. This is no longer a problem, and I obtained a delightful "shell pink" cheek color from all-vegan brand Bella Mari.

Perfume is particularly tricky to purchase online. How does one truly get the sense of a scent by looking at a webpage? That's why I was excited to discover that all-vegan perfume company Pinrose offers a "starter kit" for $9 that includes samples of all twelve of its scents.

Some other vegan makeup companies that offer their products online include Elixery, which has carefully crafted lipsticks in luxurious colors; Modern Minerals, with lovely lip glosses and eye shadows in subtle shades; Glamour Dolls, with fun and sexy colors; and Obsessive Compulsive Cosmetics, famous for their glossy lip tars in bold hues.

In addition to the many companies that offer makeup for sale at their own websites, all-vegan makeup brands such as Emani and Pacifica can be purchased online from Target, as well.

When it comes to vegan makeup, a little research can go a long way. With some preparation before shopping, you can enter stores confident that you'll find vegan products. And if you don't find what you want, you can put together just about any look by shopping online. For those of us who wear makeup, there is a big wonderful world of vegan cosmetics available to us.

Vegan and Vegan-Friendly Makeup Companies

When I went vegan, I was thrilled to find a few makeup companies that offered high-quality vegan options. Today, there are many vegan and vegan-friendly brands to choose from. These companies produce products in colors ranging from subtle hues, like the reasonably priced offerings from Everyday Minerals, to supernatural shades such as Lime Crime's sparkling metallic Lawn/Flamingo eye shadow duo in pink and green.

Below are lists of some of the all-vegan and vegan-friendly makeup brands on the market today. None of these companies test on animals. Remember, ingredients change, so you'll want to check company websites for updates.

Vegan	Vegan-Friendly (Many, but not all, products are vegan)
Arbonne	Ecco Bella
Aromi	E.L.F.
Au Naturale	Hourglass
Axiology	Kat Von D
Beauty Without Cruelty	Lush
Blackbird Cosmetics	Nars
Black Moon Cosmetics	Too Faced
Colorevolution	Urban Decay
Color Me Chad	Young blood
Concrete Minerals	
Earthly Body	
Elixery	
Emani	
Everyday Minerals	
FiOR Minerals	
Geek Chic Cosmetics	
Glamour Dolls	
INIKA	
Lime Crime	
LunatiCK	
Modern Minerals	
Obsessive Compulsive Cosmetics	
Overall Beauty Minerals	
Pacifica	
Red Apple Lipstick	
Root	
Strobe Cosmetics	
Terre Mere Cosmetics	
ZuZu Luxe	

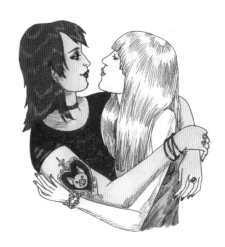

CHAPTER 4

Omnivore Dilemma: To Date or Not to Date . . . a Meat-Eater

Looking for love as a vegan, we may find ourselves wondering if we should consider dating meat-eaters or stay with those who share our lifestyle. Though some will opt to exclusively date vegans, many women who follow a cruelty-free lifestyle have found happiness with an omnivore. Often, those meat-eaters become inspired to start making more compassionate choices. Though some omnivores are more vegan-friendly than others, there are plenty of non-vegans who respect and admire us cruelty-free gals.

The Omnivore That Got Away

I went to college in the scenic Hudson Valley, at a very liberal liberal arts school called Bard. There were many artists, free thinkers, wanderers, partiers, innovators, and creative dressers. There were also a fair number of vegetarians, but I wasn't one of them. I was still in my omnivore days. I wouldn't stop eating animals until well into my thirties.

I had many crushes on creatively dressed free-thinking wandering artistic innovative partying men at Bard, some of which were requited, and some that were not.

One unrequited crush in particular baffled me for years. He was a beautiful dancer. He was tall, talented, and charming. We became friendly and though I perceived him to be possibly interested in me, my insecurities and fears kept me from pursuing the situation further. During one summer break when we were both in New York City, he called me numerous times to hang out, and we did. I still felt paralyzed by fears of inadequacy and rejection, even as we lay on the bed at his uncle's apartment, watching a movie. Sitting together in a bar, a stranger came up to tell us that we made a beautiful couple. He departed New York soon after and a relationship never became a reality. I continued to admire his beauty when we went back to Bard in the fall, while remaining deep in insecurity and fear. A big question mark hung over my head about why the relationship had never happened.

Fast-forward more than a decade to the 2000s when there was a surge of online reconnection with old friends and when I was newly vegetarian. Being single and curious, I (like many others) sought out past crushes on social networking sites. Of course the beautiful dancer was one of them. To my shock and chagrin, his username on this particular website celebrated meat. He actually had the word *meat* in his online name. *Ew*, I thought. I tried to be accepting but felt sadness. It wasn't just that he was clearly a meat-eater; it was that he was proactively endorsing and advertising the consumption of meat. Still I sent him a message. I mean, come on, he was my college crush. The conversation didn't go anywhere, and I could never get past the carnivore-a-rama aspect of his profile page.

Years passed and there was a mass movement from one social networking website to another. Remembering the experience from the last site, I, now vegan, refrained from connecting with the beautiful dancer again. But, eventually, I caved. I quickly learned that he had become a chef, and his page was littered with photographs of . . . meat. It was filled with images of carefully prepared and positioned slabs of dead animals. The warmth I still held in my heart for him was quickly cut off by a cement wall rising up in the face of the photographs. I couldn't help it. I couldn't rationalize my way out of it. It was a deep and undeniable physical and emotional reaction.

The crush rush is intense. That high feeling you may get when you see even just a photograph of someone you have feelings for can be hard to deny. But even in the face of that intense rush of warm emotion at the thought of connecting with my crush, my feelings about animals losing their lives were stronger. It's not that I thought, *I cannot connect with someone who promotes the consumption of animals*; it's that I had a powerful emotional reaction to the abundance of meat on his page. That emotional reaction overrode any lingering feelings of "crushdom." I couldn't connect with him anymore. And the big question mark of why we had never been a couple started to fade.

Reading about the plight of farmed animals opened my eyes, and helping the animals on a daily basis just by virtue of the food choices I make has dramatically impacted my life for the better. It has changed me on a deep level. Even though scrolling through the photos on my former crush's page brought up difficult feelings, I'm so grateful to be living in the reality now, instead of the disconnect.

When I was in college I couldn't understand why the beautiful dancer and I weren't dating and deeply in love. I felt confused and insecure and rejected. But as has been the case so far in my life, the universe kept me away from the totally wrong person for me, even when I demanded otherwise, crying and moping when I didn't get what I wanted. Clearly this particular crush and I were on different paths, and the fact that we never paired up seems to have been a blessing.

Looking at his profiles, I concluded that he would never consider dating a vegan, like me, in the same way that I wouldn't want to be involved with such a passionate meat-eater. When I started to work on this book, I decided to see if that conclusion was correct. I sent him a message to find out if he had or would ever consider dating someone who was vegan or vegetarian. He quickly responded, "Me dating a vegetarian would be like a porpoise dating a porcupine; on their own they are harmless, but together . . . chaos."

But then he thought further, and added, "Actually I dated a vegetarian once. I didn't push them to eat what I ate and vice versa."

I realized the beautiful dancer was perfectly open to a relationship with someone who didn't eat meat; it was I who had rejected the thought of being with someone who promoted its consumption so whole-heartedly. Suddenly, I was grateful we had never dated. I wondered, though, if there were more vegan-friendly omnivores out there.

At a party I attended recently, I met Austin, a handsome, kind, thirty-eight-year-old single omnivore man. Though I was in a committed relationship, I was curious if he would consider dating a vegan. A fitness professional and designer, he enthusiastically began to tell me about a date he had been on with a vegan woman, smiling at the memory of what was clearly an enjoyable evening for him.

Austin told me, "I like to eat everything, but I love vegan food." He tries to eat at least one vegan meal a day, and he explained that before he ventured down his current career path, he was seriously considering becoming a vegan chef. "I love the food, I think it's beautiful." He said he finds it "very attractive, if someone wants to eat that way."

Austin filled me in on his recent date with the vegan woman. The two simply fell into a conversation with each other while walking side by side on a New York City sidewalk. "We just smiled at each other and started talking . . . She said, 'You've got really great energy.'"

"I was a little surprised," Austin confided, of finding out that his lovely new acquaintance was vegan. "I don't think I've ever dated somebody who was vegan before."

Taking things a step further with the woman, Austin suggested one of New York City's most elegant and established plant-based restaurants, Candle 79, for dinner. "I want you to be happy," he told her. The two had a wonderful dinner, with neither feeling deprived or diminished due to their dietary differences.

I asked Austin if he would go out with another vegan woman after the experience with his first vegan date. "Yeah," he said without hesitation, "I'd marry a vegan woman."

Clearly Austin not only accepts the vegan lifestyle, but he also appreciates and admires it. He is a vegan-friendly omnivore who thinks that living a vegan lifestyle is "beautiful."

Though there may be some omnivores who we choose not to date, there are many vegan women who find true love with non-vegans. Austin is a good-looking, yoga-teaching, friendly, positive single person who thinks it would be great to have a vegan partner. He is just one omnivore whose heart is wide open to dating vegan women. Even the beautiful dancer, with his obvious love of meat, was open to a relationship with someone who didn't eat it. He just wasn't the match for me.

You never know who's out there on the Internet or walking on the sidewalk next to you. Someone who may not be exactly like you may be exactly the right person for you.

Quiz: Could an Omnivore Be the One for Me?

Anyone who holds their values close to their heart will want to take them into consideration when dating. Most of us have certain beliefs at the core of our beings. For some, they are religious views, for others they are strong work ethics, and for those choosing veganism—we often have powerful feelings about the treatment of animals. Part of playing the dating game is staying aware of our feelings in the company of those with different values. Dating an omnivore can be a great way to expose someone unfamiliar with veganism to the issues, but only if we feel comfortable being involved with that person. Could an omnivore be the one for you? Here are some questions you can ask yourself to find out.

Questions

1) If your dinner date ordered a dish containing meat, could you still enjoy your meal?
2) Are you comfortable explaining why you are vegan, and talking about the related issues in a calm and friendly manner?

3) Do you enjoy sharing what you love about veganism with others, such as going with them to a farm animal sanctuary or cooking them a great vegan meal?

4) Do you feel secure speaking up for your vegan needs in a restaurant or store even though your partner may not understand why they are requirements?

5) Would you be able to sleep comfortably in a home that had animal products in it?

Answers:

How many questions did you answer Yes to?

0–1: You may still want to try dating an omnivore or two, but if spending time with them is painful, it might be time to seek out a fellow vegan.

2–3: It's quite possible that you can find an omnivore match. You may warm up to them if they start to express an interest in veganism, or begin to make more compassionate choices. If you never reach the comfort zone, feel free to move on.

4–5: You are such an omnivore lover! You may be exactly the person an omnivore out there is looking for. Their love for you could open their heart to veganism. Being your compassionate self may be just the inspiration they need to live a cruelty-free life.

Dating Stories: Opposites Attract?

Many vegan women dream of finding the perfect vegan partner so that they can live together in vegan harmony, but many have also found joyous and fulfilling lives with omnivores.

One woman I spoke with said that, despite wanting to only date other vegans, she was unable to find a good match who eschewed animal products. Deciding to date omnivores, she soon met a man who became her long-term love. Now he is making more compassionate choices when it comes to what he eats, a change that may not have happened if she hadn't exposed him to veganism. Because of her open-mindedness, there is less cruelty in the world.

Often vegan women see their meat-eating dates and partners begin to move toward a cruelty-free lifestyle. By opening your heart to omnivores, you may find love and could inspire someone else to live more compassionately.

Living Life With Passion and Compassion
Danielle Legg, Licensed Veterinary Technician, Health and Fitness Coach

There is something undeniably pixie-esque about thirty-something vegan Danielle Legg. Not only because of her signature "pixie" haircut, but because she has an effervescent personality and unique sense of style that are both inviting and playful. Often found in a colorful sundress, Danielle's clothes reflect her bright outlook, attracting us like bees to a beautiful flower. I first met Danielle at Farm Sanctuary's Watkins Glen shelter for rescued animals, her love of animals and commitment to veganism radiating in her glowing face and near-constant smile.

After moving from upstate New York to New York City, Danielle became a powerful presence in the metropolis's thriving vegan community. She has worked professionally and as a volunteer for numerous animal-related causes and projects, investing her energy in endeavors she truly believes in and that reflect who she is deep-down inside: a person who wants to improve the lives of animals.

Danielle didn't just grow up in an omnivorous household; she lived on a farm with cows, pigs, chickens, turkeys, sheep, and goats who were raised to be food. "I grew up eating the animals I played with," she explains. "My parents had parties where people would come over and kill our chickens and turkeys."

In her twenties, Danielle began to learn about the cruel treatment of animals raised for food on industrialized farms and those used in performances. The catalyst that sent Danielle into the realm of veganism was watching a video of the abuse endured by chickens on a factory farm. "At my core, I was horrified at what these people were doing to the chickens . . . men grabbing the animals by their legs and swinging them, or swinging them by their heads," she recounts.

"At that time, I decided I wasn't eating meat anymore. Three days later, I decided I wasn't going to have dairy or eggs," says Danielle, who was just under thirty years old at the time. Soon after, she cleared all of the animal products out of her closet, committing to a fully vegan lifestyle.

Before Danielle took the plunge, she was the omnivore in a relationship with a vegan. Her love interest had been encouraging her to make more compassionate decisions, but it was after she went vegan that the two became more serious in their romance.

Later, when single again, Danielle decided to only date other vegans. She says of that time: "It's nice to come home or hang out and know that you can go into the refrigerator and you're not going to see someone dead in there, or a piece of someone."

However, over time, things changed for Danielle, and a new perspective came into play. She wanted to open the door to more people. Danielle decided to include omnivores in her dating pool. She credits her vegan roommate, who dated omnivores himself, with convincing her to make the change.

In a potential partner, Danielle looks for someone she connects with. While only dating vegans, she felt that her dates were so insistent on being with someone with the same ethics that they ignored all of her other qualities. "[Veganism] is very much a large part of who I am but I am not just vegan. I like old music, and I like museums, and I'm nuts about my dog and my cat . . . It's interesting to get to know someone and kind of see who they are aside from this one big thing."

Danielle created a profile for herself on a popular dating website and included the word *vegan* in her screen name, but is staying open to dating omnivores. She received a few offensive messages, taking her to task on her ethical lifestyle. Danielle ignored those and found herself connecting with someone who shared her love of a local "dive" restaurant next to her apartment building. The two began dating, and this particular person turned out to be an omnivore who respected her cruelty-free lifestyle. Although he's not vegan, now that Danielle has introduced him to great plant-based foods, he makes requests to go to his favorite vegan restaurants. He also asks her a steady stream of questions about animal rights issues.

When talking about such serious subject matter, Danielle says, "I'm with him like I am with anyone else—always pleasant, always happy, always smiling and happy to give the information." Now her open-minded omnivore has his own personal vegan ambassador.

Because of Danielle's open heart, this particular meat-eater is now exploring veganism. The omnivore in her life has an opportunity to see animals through Danielle's loving and compassionate eyes. Danielle has let her vegan light shine, and now that light is shining on someone else.

Vegan and Omnivore Meet Midway
Sarah Gross, Founder and President of Rescue Chocolate and Producer of the New York City, Arizona, and California Vegetarian Food Festivals

I met Sarah Gross for the first time when we were seated around a table with other New York City vegans, planning the launch of a new animal rights nonprofit organization. Sarah is the founder of Rescue Chocolate, a vegan chocolate company that donates all of its net profits to animal rescue organizations around the United States. She also co-organizes the massive annual New York City, Arizona, and California Vegetarian Food Festivals as well as the Better Booze Festival.

Sarah remembers two major shifts that happened in her life when she went vegan, more than fifteen years ago. She suddenly had more energy than her peers, and she began to enjoy her food more. "I think (and there are studies backing me up), that one's palate shifts, and tastes become more intense when one isn't eating animal products. I love and look forward to food so much more now than I ever did in my pre-vegan days . . . The energy bit makes sense as your body's not wasting any energy breaking down animal muscle," says Sarah.

The suitors who Sarah considered dating rarely took her to task about her compassionate lifestyle. Only one person voiced any kind of concern or objection to her veganism. The dating prospect, who Sarah had met online, flat out refused to go out with her once she shared with him that she was vegan. "This isn't going to work out," he said, cutting their discourse short. Perhaps he saved her the trouble of spending time with someone who was unable to accept her for who she was. It seems this missed connection would have been a mismatch if brought to fruition. By being true to herself and honest with others, Sarah followed her path into more agreeable territory.

When Sarah met her now-husband, he was a no-holds-barred, 100 percent omnivore. She has never dated vegans exclusively and knew about his all-inclusive diet before they became involved. She says, "There was no conflict. I always take people for who they are."

Sarah has never actively worked to convert her husband, Paolo, to veganism, but makes an effort to set a good example by "trying to make my food smell as good and look as appetizing as possible . . . I also put on vegetarian-focused events regularly, and he'll attend all of those, nibbling at bites and listening to the evening's animal or vegan-focused speaker," she says.

Though Sarah never expected or demanded a shift, by following what she knows is right for herself, she has seen her guy slowly move toward a more plant-based diet, and that has brought her more happiness. Two events in particular saw him make significant changes: the first, watching Farm Sanctuary president and cofounder Gene Baur speaking about veganism on television, and the second, the loss of a close relative to cancer. "He flew to be with her for the last week of her life and got a really visceral, physical wakeup call about life and one's health," she explains. The experience motivated Paolo to commit to eating vegan dinners several nights a week. He also began participating in Meatless Mondays, abstaining from eating meat for one full day a week. Sarah stresses that this move toward a vegan diet was a huge step for someone who she had met years before as an unapologetic omnivore.

By being herself, and following her heart, Sarah has not only inspired the thousands of people who attend her events, but she has seen the person she loves make compassionate changes in his own life.

Sarah's advice for vegan ladies who are dating is: "Respect the person you're seeing for who he is. Starting out a relationship by immediately trying to make someone live your lifestyle isn't going to work, in most cases.

You need to fully understand where he's coming from and let things progress naturally. If he's empathetic to your choices and respects them, this is someone worth pursuing."

Computing Her Options
Grace Sullivan, Psychiatric Social Worker

In Grace, gentleness and confidence combine in such an inviting way that when I sit down to talk to her, I want to stay there for hours. She also possesses a sly sense of humor that comes out from time to time, reminding me that though veganism is serious business, it's important to have fun in life. It's no surprise to me that she is a successful psychiatric social worker since speaking with her is therapeutic.

Grace, who lives in New York City, went vegetarian in her late twenties and fully vegan at thirty-four. A veteran of two long-term relationships (with omnivores), she is now back in the swing of meeting new partner possibilities—utilizing the technology of online dating services.

Grace is completely comfortable going out with omnivores. "I understand how people who aren't horrible people eat meat . . . I have many friends and family members who eat animals and I still care about them," she says, adding that a like-minded vegan isn't necessarily going to be a good match in other important areas. "Just because someone's vegan, it doesn't mean that I'm attracted to them or we have anything else in common, or that they're not racist, or homophobic, or anti-Semitic. I've met vegans who are all of those things and that's actually far more intolerable," she says.

As far as dating omnivores, Grace says, "I think there's something to be said for educating people when they're in my life . . ." Grace takes dates with meat-eaters as opportunities to teach them about the realities of farming animals and the benefits of vegan living. As a direct result, some of those she has engaged with have moved toward a more cruelty-free existence. "I've had people who told me . . . though they didn't go vegan, they were a lot more conscious about how they ate, and what they ate, and they had really decreased their animal product consumption. And were continuing to do so after we stopped dating." Though dating omnivores may not be comfortable for all vegans, Grace followed what was best for her, and by doing so inspired some dates to eat more kindly. By being true to herself, she decreased the amount of suffering in the world.

When speaking with non-vegans about the issues, Grace tries not to bombard them, but share in a gentle manner. "There's an idea of the angry, strident vegan . . . we have lots to be angry about, but there's something to be said for communicating with people in a way that allows them to hear you." For instance, Grace refrains from speaking about the gorier details of the egg industry over dinner, choosing a more opportune moment to fully educate someone who has expressed interest.

Though Grace is perfectly willing to spend time with a non-vegan, she adds that for her to consider someone as a partner, "they have to be pro-vegan . . . They have to really support it." She recently took one such supportive omnivore date to Brooklyn vegan restaurant Champs and "he ordered the 'vegan slam,'" she says, "and ate every last bite of tofu scramble, tempeh bacon, and 'soysage.' I was very impressed."

Grace is open and up-front about her veganism in her online dating profiles. "If they're going to be put off that I'm vegan then they might as well be put off right away . . ."

The results have been mixed. One person who advertised in his profile that he would not date a vegan missed Grace's mention and contacted her. When she pointed out this detail to him, he said, ". . . I actually really admire your life choice and I think it's really impressive." Though their exchange didn't end in wedding bells, Grace's openness and honesty about her ethical choices led to a positive and heartfelt communication with someone who had previously shut the door on vegans. She expressed who she was in a kind way, and another person took a second look at their negative views of veganism.

Grace advises, "Don't let [being vegan] hold you back, the fear of, *Oh, God, no one's going to want to go out with . . . a vegan.*" She adds, "You never know what it is people are going to like or dislike." Grace also encourages women to speak up for their vegan requirements, pointing out that sometimes, as women, "we are less likely to ask for our needs to be met, we don't want to be a problem." She says, "It's okay to just politely ask . . ." If the person you are dating finds it too challenging, maybe they're not the right person for you.

Grace also suggests showing dates that veganism isn't all about saying no by baking a batch of delicious vegan cookies. "Dessert activism is very successful in my experience," she says.

Excellent vegan restaurants, cakes, cookies—and most of all the fabulous person that you are—are all great ways to show an omnivore how amazing vegan living can be.

You Do You and I'll Do Me
Tracy Habenicht, Works for an Animal Rights Organization

With her quiet level-headedness, it's easy to listen to Tracy, whether you are an omnivore or a vegan. She brings her love of animals into both her personal and professional lives, living a cruelty-free lifestyle and working for an international animal rights organization that advocates for veganism. Tracy has found a lot of peace in the acceptance of her current and past partners' omnivorous diets. Once married to a meat-eater and now dating one, Tracy opts to live her life according to her ethics and not try to change the choices of the person she is involved with.

Tracy first went vegetarian in 2006 after reading online that pigs were smarter than three-year-old children. "I had a niece at the time who was two and I thought she was a genius, and if pigs are smarter than she was, I couldn't eat them anymore." She became vegan soon after in August 2007.

Tracy was dating an omnivore at the time, who she eventually married and later divorced, though their dietary differences were not the reason for the breakup. "I . . . realize that people are on their own path and they change when they want to change, and I can't force that," she says.

When the couple went their separate ways, Tracy continued to keep her heart open to omnivores. "I didn't ask myself if I wanted to date vegans or vegetarians, maybe because I had already been married to an omnivore . . . and it wasn't an issue for me." Her new boyfriend is a meat-eater who loves to cook fantastic vegan food for the both of them.

Though Tracy worried that her veganism might pose a problem in her new relationship, it turned out to be a non-issue. Her beau is respectful of her lifestyle, and all is well in this mixed match.

Says Tracy, "I don't want to change him. In relationships, in general, it's impossible to change people." She adds, "It's going really well."

"It's so difficult to find someone to date and to be with," says Tracy, "if you put a limitation on it—they have to be vegan—then it just makes it even more difficult. However, for some people it will become a major disagreement in their relationship . . . [K]now yourself and know what you can deal with and just go from there in choosing who to date." In staying open to others, but true to herself, Tracy has found a partner who supports her and her compassionate lifestyle.

Love and Legumes in the South
Katy G., Montessori Teacher

From the moment Katy picks up the phone for our interview, I'm swept up in her fun, funny, tell-it-like-it-is attitude and subtle southern twang. With her honest and humorous manner, she shares a wealth of experiences and knowledge about veganism, making it clear that abstaining from animal products is simply common sense.

Though ethical reasons initially drove Katy, who lives in Decatur, Georgia, to go vegetarian, she dropped dairy from her diet to help her allergies. "I felt so bad every year. I was on allergy shots . . . I couldn't breathe and I was just miserable," she says. After hearing that giving up dairy might help her to feel better, she stopped consuming it. The improvement was immense: "It did not take two weeks for it to make an enormous difference," she says. "I felt like a different person." Seeing her body respond in such an obvious way, Katy decided to take the opportunity to fully commit to veganism. She explains, "I had been thinking about going vegan anyway," and decided, "it's better for the environment and it's better for the animals, so I'll just stay vegan." She has now been vegan for fifteen years.

Katy met her current boyfriend while out to see a band play, "which is where I meet everyone," she shares. Though he's an omnivore, he's supportive of Katy's veganism, and often prepares food for both of them. "Luckily for me, he's the kind of person who loves to cook," she says. "He's not scared of tofu, and he's fine making vegan food." The couple can often be found cooking together in the kitchen. "It's one of my favorite things we do," says Katy.

Although she has tried, Katy has never dated a vegan. She explains that the last time that she was single, she set out to date only other vegans, but couldn't find any who would be a good match for her. She went to vegan potlucks and a book signing by vegan cookbook author Isa Chandra Moskowitz that was "slam-packed with vegans," but walked away without a mate. So she decided to date omnivores.

Katy allows her boyfriend to bring meat into her home, but she doesn't prepare or eat it. "I live in the real world," she says, "where you have to be around people who eat meat, and . . . it's not my favorite, I don't wanna cook it, and I don't wanna be around it all the time . . . but . . . you have to be around it, so it's okay."

Often cooking outside, grilling is a major consideration. Katy solves the problem of her boyfriend cooking meat at the same time she prepares her food by having a two-tiered grill—with her items on the top shelf, and her boyfriend's below. That way her vegan food stays clear of any undesirable drippings.

Katy doesn't actively attempt to veganize her current partner, but they do talk about related issues. "I don't think right now he'd want to make a change, I mean, he knows dairy is not so healthy for you. He knows meat's not the healthiest choice . . . if he ever made a serious decision to fully go vegan it would probably be for health reasons. But he loves dogs . . . I did bring up speciesism . . . certain animals you eat, certain animals you buy 'em crazy outfits and parade 'em around. If you guys all want to eat animals, why aren't you eating dogs and cats? I don't understand it."

Though Katy's boyfriend has the option of eating meat at her house, he has been consuming less and less of it. As with other vegans dating omnivores, by living according to her own standards, taking actions in response to her ethics, and passing on information without pressuring her partner, Katy's boyfriend has reduced the cruelty in his diet.

Everything is fine at home when it comes to the hybrid household, but when spending time with her partner's family, Katy has found the dynamics to be not as simple. Arriving during the setup stage of one of his family's events, she discovered the offerings to be, "Sausage dip, brisket, some other kind of meat in another crockpot, a bunch of cheeses . . . it was like, meatastic." Spending the weekend with her beau's relatives, Katy struggled to find food to eat. In the end, she says, "It was fine," but adds, "I think next time . . . if we're going anywhere where it's 'his people,' I'm going to say, 'Can you let 'em know I'm vegan?' before we go there."

Katy has personally experienced the great health improvements that a vegan diet can bring. She is strong and surefooted in her convictions, yet accepts that her boyfriend may not hold the same beliefs. Together they have found peaceful coexistence despite their dietary divide.

Vegan Meets Omnivore, Magic Ensues
Allison Laakko, Fine Artist
Josh Malerman, Author and Musician

Artist Allison Laakko lives with her fiancé, Josh Malerman (author of the internationally popular novel *Bird Box*), in Royal Oak, Michigan. Together their home is a hub of creativity with Josh churning out one horror story after another (in addition to fronting the band The High Strung) and Allison creating a spectrum of art projects.

Having grown up in a small town in Michigan's Upper Peninsula, Allison's family were very "nature-oriented people who loved everything outdoors and were very self-reliant in terms of food," she says. "They have always had large gardens with almost every vegetable you can think of . . . My mom had been a vegetarian for a greater portion of her life." With this nature-centric start, choosing a vegan path felt close to home for Allison.

"My own health and well-being [were] the primary reason[s] I wanted to cut out animal products, but it didn't happen entirely until I did more research on what the consumption of animal products was doing to the world around me. Obviously the treatment of animals used for consumption is a horrible problem," Allison says, adding, "Many of the environmental harms the earth faces can be directly linked to the factory farming and food production industries."

The couple found love when Allison unexpectedly ended up at a nightclub where Josh's band was performing. They briefly met, but no numbers were exchanged. The magic they felt was mutual, though, and thanks to a social networking website, they soon reconnected. "We've basically been attached at the hip ever since," says smitten Allison.

Allison filled in Josh (an omnivore) about her vegan lifestyle early on. She says, "I think when a person is very health-conscious, it's just one of those things that come up right away in conversation. When he asked to take me out to eat, he quickly learned about my favorite restaurant, Cacao Café, a vegan raw food joint. He took me there as often as I wanted, and it ended up being one of his favorite spots as well . . ."

Josh was excited to learn all about Allison, including the veganism that was clearly important to her. She explained the cruelty of animal farming and its harms to the environment when they were first getting to know each other. Josh was intrigued. "When she talks to you," he explains, ". . . she has so much information to back up why it's healthy, and why this is a wise choice . . ." He adds that he never felt as if Allison was pressuring him when she was sharing her reasons to be vegan: "It's done in this very intelligent way, where you almost cannot argue against it." Not only was Josh interested in Allison's ethical lifestyle, but he saw it as one of her most admirable traits.

By following her own cruelty-free and healthy path, and explaining her reasons, Allison inspired her beloved to eat a more plant-based diet. "Josh was a big meat-eater before me, but it wasn't necessarily because he just absolutely loved meat, it was more that that's just what he knew and what he was used to," she explains.

While eating healthy, meat-free food with Allison, Josh began to see changes in himself. "He said he could feel the difference in how he felt after a fresh vegetarian or vegan meal right away, in terms of just feeling more energized and lighter, instead of feeling heavy and bloated . . . After eating a healthier, more plant-based diet for a few weeks, he was feeling lighter and healthier all the time . . . His diet has been more plant-based ever since," says Allison.

Josh, who now eats few animal products, explains that he sees veganism as "one of those behind-the-curtain moments, where once you see that it's feasible, possible, even healthy, even healthier, better for the environment—once you see all these things, how do you un-see those?" He has welcomed the lifting of guilty feelings as a result of dramatically reducing the cruelty in his diet. Now not only is Josh eating much more humanely, but he enjoys introducing omnivore friends and family to delicious cruelty-free foods.

Josh explains that Allison's great health and abundant energy helped inspire him to move in the plant-based direction: "Here's this person that is like insanely fit, and healthy, who runs marathons, who's vegan." Allison dispelled any myths for him that vegans might be lethargic or short on protein.

A few animal products stay in the refrigerator for Josh, but this has not caused any conflict for the couple. Both are comfortable living in a mostly-vegan household. Neither has had to negate who they are to accommodate the other.

Allison didn't seek to manipulate Josh to do what she wanted. It was her great example, her gentle sharing of information, and Josh's own experience of feeling better physically and emotionally, that led him to lessen his consumption of animal products.

"I truly believe that a vegan diet is the right way to eat, but just like any other belief system, I don't discriminate when someone doesn't feel this way," says Allison, adding, "Now just think of what a pity it would be, what an awful shame, had I passed up on Josh because I found out our diets were different, and just never gave it a chance. I'd have missed out on the love of my life, the love of the millennium!"

Lending Library: Movies and Books to Share With Your Omnivore

Is your omnivore partner (or potential mate) asking questions about veganism? Is the person you adore curious about your cruelty-free philosophy? Has he or she started to eat more plant-based foods when they are around you? A great way to nurture a budding interest in compassionate living is to share some of your movies and books about the issues. Don't have any favorites of your own? Here are some that may fit the bill.

Movies

Babe (1995), directed by Chris Noonan

Pig meets dog meets farmer in this fictional film about believing in oneself, and in others, and not subscribing to cliché beliefs about farm animals.

Cowspiracy (2014), directed by Kip Andersen and Keegan Kuhn

A documentary that digs deep in an attempt to uncover why leading environmental organizations aren't addressing the massive negative impact of animal farming on the planet.

Earthlings (2005), directed by Shaun Monson

A stunning documentary film that looks at the suffering animals endure around the world for the sake of varied industries.

Food, Inc. (2008), directed by Robert Kenner

This documentary takes a close look at the ills of corporate farming, including the extensive and often hidden abuses of animals.

Forks Over Knives (2011), directed by Lee Fulkerson

Looking closely at groundbreaking research by T. Colin Campbell, PhD and Caldwell B. Esselstyn Jr., MD, this film reveals the negative impact of eating animal products on people's health and the benefits of a plant-based diet.

The Ghosts in Our Machine (2013), directed by Liz Marshall

Liz Marshall's film focuses on the work of photographer Jo-Anne McArthur, who travels around the world documenting the animals who have fallen victim to industry and those who have been rescued. This documentary is an account of egregious cruelty and a tribute to those who have fallen victim to it.

Vegucated (2011), directed by Marisa Miller Wolfson

A fun, lighthearted documentary (that tackles some serious issues) about three New Yorkers trying out a vegan diet for six weeks. We met writer, director, and editor Marisa Miller Wolfson in chapter 1.

Books
The 30-Day Vegan Challenge (2014), by Colleen Patrick-Goudreau

It's no secret that I am a huge fan of Colleen Patrick-Goudreau (whom we'll meet in chapter 8) and her *Food for Thought* podcast. In this book, Goudreau offers a guide for beginners who want to try out a vegan diet.

The China Study (2006), by T. Colin Campbell, PhD and Thomas M. Campbell II, MD

For those seeking concrete facts about the health benefits of cutting animal products out of their diet, this book offers scientific data that even a skeptical omnivore can appreciate. I studied it when I was going through cancer treatments and the content completely convinced me that a plant-based diet was a critical component in my recovery and maintenance of good health.

Do Unto Animals (2015), by Tracey Stewart

Do Unto Animals is a great book for the omnivore who is looking to improve their relationship with animals. This #1 *New York Times* bestseller opens the door to the emotional connection between human and non-human animals.

What a Fish Knows (2016), by Jonathan Balcombe

Jonathan Balcombe has written a number of books that explore the emotional lives of animals. In this one, he shares that the inner worlds of aquatic beings may be much more complex than we assume.

Living the Farm Sanctuary Life (2015), by Gene Baur with Gene Stone

Written by Farm Sanctuary president and cofounder Gene Baur and coauthor Gene Stone, this book includes a wealth of information about how to live a life with less cruelty, lots of recipes, and useful tips that will help beginners learn more about veganism.

Main Street Vegan (2012), by Victoria Moran with Adair Moran

Victoria Moran is a vegan superhero of sorts, writing books and speaking to large audiences on the topic, as well as teaching her popular Main Street Vegan Academy course. In this book, she offers new vegans great support, giving them the resources they need to embrace a compassionate lifestyle.

Running, Eating, Thinking (2014), edited by Martin Rowe

The perfect loaner for an athlete who doesn't believe they will get adequate nutrition if they go vegan. This philosophical book collects essays by fifteen vegan runners.

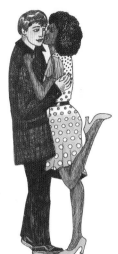

CHAPTER 5

Two of a Kind: Dating and Partnering With Other Vegans

Vegan women may take different paths to partnering with another vegan. Some dive into a relationship with an omnivore who later cuts out the cruelty. Some fall in love with a person who just happens to be vegan. And in some cases, a couple will go vegan together.

Some of us vegans consider ourselves to be "vegansexuals," a person who will only enter into a relationship with another vegan. Though this may seem like a modern concept, the idea has been around for a long time. Author Mary Shelley depicted the monster in *Frankenstein* as a vegansexual. In the book, the character explains, "I do not destroy the lamb and the kid to glut my appetite; acorns and berries afford me sufficient nourishment. My companion will be of the same nature as myself, and will be content with the same fare."

Whether one is a vegansexual or just happens to land in a relationship with someone else living a cruelty-free lifestyle, there are many benefits to coupling with a fellow vegan. Women I spoke with enjoyed having a cruelty-free kitchen, a more united front at family events, and someone to share the excitement of new vegan products with as just some of the advantages.

Though many omnivore partners eventually move toward a compassionate lifestyle, if you simply cannot tolerate sitting across the table from a date who is eating an animal, you may want to consider dating another vegan.

My Vegan Love

Upon entering the dating game as a vegan, I never stopped to think, *Do I only want to date vegans, or would I be okay partnering with an omnivore?* If I had, I probably would have been thrown by thoughts such as, *What do I do if an omnivore partner wants to keep eggs in the refrigerator?* Or, *What would I do if he wanted to raise our children as meat-eaters?*

Luckily my lack of over-thinking led me to exactly the right place. I made no black-and-white decisions about whether to date non-vegans, but by simply following what felt right, I ended up with someone who went vegan days after we began seeing each other. A vegetarian for decades, my guy asked me why I was vegan over one of our first lunches. I calmly and matter-of-factly told him what had prompted me to cut out dairy, and he decided to go vegan, just like that. I had no prepared speech, I didn't lecture him for half an hour, I just told him the truth, and he responded. And the truth is something that is very important to me. So by being honest with myself and with the person who was sitting across from me, I not only found a fellow vegan, but someone who also valued the truth. Someone who didn't want to be part of a system that sees newborn calves torn away from their moms and slaughtered for veal.

Living now with that same fellow vegan, it's hard to imagine sharing a home with someone who doesn't have those ethical commitments. I still have plenty of omnivore friends and family, but when I shut the door and take my animal-free shoes off, I want to know that I am in a safe space where my core values are not violated.

I never guessed that this is where I'd end up. I've been interested in vegans and omnivores alike. As a dater, I didn't discriminate against non-vegans, I just followed my own path and landed where I was happy. And that turned out to be with another person who shared my ethics concerning animals.

What I have learned from living and being in a relationship with a partner who is vegan is that I am grateful not to open the refrigerator door and see the carcasses of chickens. I am grateful not to have to explain why I don't want a down blanket (the result of unnecessary cruelty to birds). I am grateful that my suggestions of going to vegan restaurants are met with enthusiasm. I am grateful to have wonderful days at farm animal sanctuaries with my partner—knowing we aren't going to be hurting the animals we are embracing when we return home. I am grateful that the meals that I cook are met with grins and not grimaces. I am grateful that when we visit our families, we are a team with requests based on our values instead of one person trying to defend their lifestyle.

While staying at my family's house in Connecticut during the holiday season, I opened the refrigerator to find a giant turkey carcass. I have spoken to other people who have experienced what I have since going vegan—of no longer perceiving the bodies of dead animals as food, but seeing them as living beings who have died. The body didn't look like food to me; it looked like the remains of someone who had once been a majestic bird, probably kept in terrible conditions, with the tip of his beak seared off, never getting to enjoy the sun, or the grass beneath his feet. The one moment that the remains of the bird spent in my field of vision brought up a cluster of feelings ranging from shock to sadness to anger. The fun and comfort of being with my family for the holidays was breached by the trauma of seeing a dead body in the refrigerator. I was angry that this beautiful bird had lost his life and was so perfunctorily placed on a shelf, to be eaten. That he had been killed because of a holiday tradition, dying for no other reason than so many other turkeys had been killed for the same event previously. The death of an animal is not necessary for our nourishment, and definitely not a requirement to celebrate a joyous time of year. I closed the door and left the kitchen. I hated knowing the body sat in the other room.

Perhaps if I lived with an omnivore, I'd be immune to these strong feelings about the death of a bird who was farmed to be food. But these feelings about animals who have suffered are important to me. They are part of what fuels me to keep moving forward and advocating for living beings subjected to cruel conditions. I imagine that if I were to live in a household with a partner who was eating animal products, I might shut off from those feelings. There would be no more mourning, and less of a connection with the animals. I value my emotional connection with non-human animals and want to mourn their deaths. Having been treated as commodities for their entire lives, that's the least I can offer them.

At this point, I must come fully clean: In our animal-loving home, we house three cats, who eat animals. I am aware that vegan cat food exists, but as born carnivores who require taurine (found in meat), I don't believe it is my right to deny cats their natural needs. I have heard firsthand accounts of people trying to feed their cats vegan diets and seeing them suffer the medical consequences. As a human who has the choice of whether or not to consume animals, I have chosen not to. Cats, however, do not have this choice. And as someone who has chosen to take care of three cats, I consider it my obligation to serve them food that is healthy for them. I don't enjoy feeding them; I would rather not have those cans of meat in my house, and I would prefer not to open them to see the bodies of dead animals. I feel for the animals who lost their lives to become food for cats, but this is the choice that I have made in my commitment to my feline companions. And as an imperfect vegan, this is probably not the only non-vegan substance in my home. I do my best. However, there is no meat in our fridge for humans. I think of the turkey who was sacrificed to be a holiday meal for my family. The death of that bird was unnecessary when there are plenty of festive plant-based food options for people. My partner and I have no need to eat an animal or any product that came from one.

I am also grateful for those who are vegans dating and living with omnivores. They are sharing their truth with those who could potentially grow from it and might become vegan themselves. Vegans who are romantically involved with omnivores are speaking up for the animals by representing the vegan lifestyle to others in the most personal of contexts. They are demonstrating unconditional love for their partners and sharing their compassionate lives.

Dating Stories: I'm Vegan, Hope You're Vegan Too

Dating another vegan can offer the comfort of knowing you and your partner see eye to eye on issues that are very near and dear to your heart. When it comes down to it, veganism is all about love: love of the animals, love of yourself, and love of the planet. Why shouldn't all of that love be part of a loving relationship with another human being?

You may find that you and someone you love are inspired to go vegan together, and it can be part of your relationship. Making that transition with a partner can offer the opportunity to discuss your opinions and actions with that person as part of your intimacy. For instance, whether to immediately discard all non-vegan clothing.

Another benefit of partnering with a fellow vegan is that you will have a like-minded mate when it comes to the holidays or raising children.

I spoke to a number of women who are greatly enjoying living in relationships with fellow vegans. Some sought to date only vegans, and some arrived in a place with a vegan partner having been open to omnivores. From not having to debate with a spouse about what to feed children, to the comfort of a home free of animal products, there are many strong arguments for partnering with another vegan. For some of us, being open to omnivores may be a way to spread the vegan love, but for others, we will be happiest sharing our lives with a vegan.

All in the (Vegan) Family
Aimee Christian, Works for an Animal Welfare Organization
Johnny Christian, Stay-at-Home Parent

Aimee can usually be found dressed in all black, with thick ebony hair, porcelain skin, and sporting a bright smile. She was my original vegan friend and she introduced me to Farm Sanctuary. In fact, the first time I visited the organization's Watkins Glen shelter for farm animals, she drove me there in her car with an open box housing a clutch of rescued baby chicks in the backseat, who chirped all the way to their new home. Aimee and I stood together and watched the young birds walk onto the dirt for the first time. It was an emotional and magical moment to see these infants step into a new life of peace and freedom.

After becoming vegetarian in high school, in her early twenties Aimee decided to try veganism for a month. She explains, ". . . I started to learn about factory farming just by kind of clicking around, and learned that the animals who live have it worse than the animals who don't . . . and that dying at six weeks is probably the best thing that could happen to a chicken . . . or dying in infancy is the best thing that could happen to a calf, rather than having to grow up basically in slavery . . ."

Aimee adds, ". . . at the end of the month I realized [being vegan] really wasn't as difficult as I thought it was going to be, so that was it." She's been happily vegan ever since.

When Aimee committed to veganism, her dietary changes were immediate, while she dealt with her wardrobe later. When she realized the time had come to let go, she says, "I went through my closet once and for all . . . [and] removed everything that was wool and silk and leather . . . I had [purchased] them used and sort of was of the mind-set that if I don't use them, then the animal died for nothing. But then it occurred to me at one point that any use of an animal product is exploitation, and it sends a message . . ."

Aimee and now-husband Johnny's romance is the stuff modern-day fairy tales are made of. He spotted her at a goth club thirteen years ago in New York City, where they both lived at the time. "I've loved her since the first day I saw her," he says.

When the soon-to-be lovebirds initially crossed paths, Aimee had already been vegan for about five years. Johnny knew about her compassionate lifestyle right off the bat.

Aimee says that when she's getting to know someone she's just met, "It's kind of like, *Hi, my name is Aimee, I'm this age, I live at this place, and I'm vegan.* You know it's kind of part of who I am, so it's not something that I ever need to sit down with somebody to have a heart-to-heart about. It just kind of comes out casually when I'm getting to know somebody."

Johnny was an omnivore, or as he explains it, "I wasn't really anything. When Aimee and I first met, I really only ate when I absolutely had to. I ate anything that was put in front of me."

Charmed as he was by Aimee, Johnny wanted to play his cards right. "I lied and told her I was vegetarian because I thought it would help my case. I didn't really understand or even care about what it meant to be vegan . . . [S]he told me she wouldn't even consider dating anyone seriously who wasn't vegan."

"It did become a deal breaker for me," says Aimee. "It's just sort of a given that another person and I would see eye to eye in this way. I can't imagine having a refrigerator that's full of animal products, even if I'm not eating them . . . I could not imagine raising a child with these conflicting ideals . . ."

Johnny admittedly went vegan "because Aimee was vegan." Soon he found that he not only loved Aimee, but he shared her love of a vegan lifestyle: ". . . the realization that I was no longer participating in harming and killing animals to eat their meat and drink their milk started to sink in and suddenly it was the only logical choice. As I stuck with it, it became a no-brainer. Living with Aimee and learning more about veganism, I realized I should have been vegan all along. Ignorance is bliss, but now that I know the truth, I will never go back."

Aimee and Johnny have now been married for six years and are raising two young children. Aimee sees many benefits when it comes to part-nering with another vegan. "We are on the same page when it comes to all of the family drama around Thanksgiving or Christmas or what [family] are serving . . . There's only one message our children are hearing . . . It's one voice, it's one philosophy, and it's how we define our home, our family, our lifestyle . . . this is how we raise our family and live our lives. It's really nice."

Lighting Up Each Other's Lives With Vegan Love
Joy Pierson, Co-Owner and Nutritionist at the Candle Restaurants
Bart Potenza, Founder of the Candle Restaurants

Joy Pierson and Bart Potenza run world-renowned vegan restaurants Candle Cafe (two locations), and Candle 79 in New York City, but are also an adoring married couple who have been together for more than two decades. Both seem to exude a similar happiness and love of life, which grow exponentially when they are around each other. It is this same sense of love that one encounters stepping into one of their establishments and eating their delicious dishes.

"Together we went vegan," says Joy. She had met her husband-to-be in 1987 when she ate the delightful vegetarian food he had prepared for her at his Healthy Candle restaurant, an earlier incarnation of today's Candle establishments. "Bart made me a sandwich and my life was never the same.

Because it made me feel so good, and it changed my life, I wanted to share it," says Joy, who soon became involved with the restaurant.

Joy and Bart were close friends for about two years before diving into a romantic relationship. Educated about veganism by clients and co-workers at Healthy Candle, the couple soon evolved into the devoted vegans they are today.

In 1993, Bart used the dates of his and Joy's birthdays to play the lottery, and won. That financial boost offered the pair the seed money to create Candle Cafe, now one of New York City's most popular vegan restaurants. But it wasn't always so packed with people.

"We opened the cafe . . . but we had no business," recalls Joy. The two went two years without being paid. "It was pretty scary, and I think it was another thing that got us closer, because we were and still are willing to go through the 'dark side.' The process never ends," says Joy.

Finally some great press and free advertising brought Candle Cafe into the light. But Joy points out that "running a restaurant takes constant work and the daily effort of us and many talented and compassionate people!" She adds, "I think Bart and I are both the kind of people that continually give 100 percent, because we are so committed to the mission, and like I say to people, I would never do the restaurant business if it wasn't a vegan restaurant. It's a very difficult business in general, and it was our commitment that actually led us into feeding people." If it weren't for the animals, and promoting healthy living, Joy and Bart might have landed in much different careers.

The couple has balanced their romantic relationship and running the Candle restaurants for more than twenty-five years now. "We often get asked, how did you do it?" comments Bart. "It's not a perfect science by any means—working through a relationship and business."

Says Joy, "It can be difficult at times, but I think that we really feel a deep respect for one another and we really respect each other's opinions." She adds, "I couldn't have done this without him."

Their common mission, of creating spectacular nutritious organic vegan food, brings them closer together, and the love that they take into their restaurants is palpable. One customer told Joy, "No one touched me, but I feel like I got a hug when I walked in the door." Joy and Bart's love of the animals, each other, and their clients flows out of their hearts and into their establishments. "Joy always said, the love is in the food, coming right out of the kitchen," says Bart.

"Our love, which was kindled over a sandwich, ignites love in others," says Joy. "We have hosted at the Candles and offsite catered many engagements, weddings, and special occasions, which adds to our love vibe."

"Our hope is that our love will continue to grow and light the way for generations to come while spreading vegan love on thick!" adds Bart.

Joy experiences veganism as expanding one's heart. "It's almost like another level of love and healing," she says. "We learn how to love more deeply."

Bart explains that the organic vegan food they consume is what helps keep them going. "When you feel good, and this food makes you feel really, really good, life happens. You just want to be in life bigger and broader and more." And when one feels good, one is more able to be a happy loving person in a relationship.

"At this stage, and I don't want to be partial," says Joy about hers and Bart's shared veganism, "but I do not think our life together would work if we did not share a common bond or mission—our life's work. We write, cook, and eat every recipe in our cookbooks together. That's a lot of sharing of our love in those three books. How could one of us not live the love of plant food and each other? It feels compassionate and passionate." She adds, "We've just grown in it together and it's part of our relationship fabric. We love creating meals together and we love shopping for food together, and we get excited about products together. It's such a fun part of our relationship." Joy points out their veganism also brings she and Bart together in their environmental activism. "Eating plants is our way of mitigating the effects of climate change—we love to vote with our forks every day."

Says Joy, "I know relationships where they have to split the refrigerator."

"The only thing we split is the last peach," adds Bart.

Romance Among the Stilettos
Erica Kubersky, Cofounder of MooShoes

Vegan fashionistas know MooShoes (a vegan shoe store with locations in New York City and Los Angeles) is the ultimate cruelty-free footwear lover's destination. Make sure not to drool on the samples as you peruse shelves and shelves of gorgeous, animal-free shoes. MooShoes was the first vegan shoe shop in New York City, opened more than a decade ago by sisters Erica and Sara Kubersky. As love would have it, Erica's husband-to-be, Justin, came in on opening day.

Says Erica: "I met him twelve years ago; he was a customer at the store . . . he came in [again] after that and we started talking, well, actually Sara asked him out for me—that's what sisters do."

Erica is soft-spoken, but always tells it like it is. Her down-to-earth attitude makes it easy to forget that she and her sister are vegan innovators who opened their New York City store long before veganism gained widespread popularity.

Justin was already vegan when the two met, but Erica didn't require that potential partners share her cruelty-free lifestyle. Though her preference was to be with another vegan, she didn't believe that narrowing the possibilities to that dating pool was a realistic option.

However, Erica shares that differing values concerning animals have always affected her relationships. "As much as I try to be open-minded, I have a hard time once somebody knows the facts," she says of those she dated who continued to consume animal products.

Erica stopped eating meat when she was only eight after spending time up close and personal with cows on a kibbutz in Israel. She recounts: "The wheels started turning in my brain . . . I asked [my parents], 'Does this mean that what I'm eating comes from this animal?' and lucky for me they were really honest about it . . ." Erica's parents were supportive of her decision to go vegetarian, and they eventually stopped eating animals themselves.

Veganism came later, when Erica was in high school, at the prompting of her sister, Sara. "It was so hard," says Erica, who did not have one other vegan friend at school. After arriving at college, though, she found a tight-knit community of fellow vegans to make tofu scramble with.

Though a shared commitment to the animals is something that Erica values greatly in her marriage, she comments, "There has to be more than that." She considers consuming animal products a simple moral issue with a very clear correct response, but she adds that veganism is not the only thing holding her and her husband together. "There definitely are aspects of our relationship that are equally important. It just goes back to the basic things—being compatible as far as humor and things we like to do," she says.

Erica had dated omnivores before meeting Justin, including one she met in college. But because of their ethical split, difficulties would often arise in the day-to-day living of their lives together. "It's hard to watch somebody eat a hamburger across from you," she says. Though he moved toward a more plant-based diet when they were together, Erica found that it was less than a sincere shift. "You think you've come so far and then in the end it turns out that they're kind of excited to get rid of you for a meal so that they can eat what they've really been wanting, and that's always so heartbreaking."

Erica never made a conscious decision to not date omnivores. She was simply honest with herself and with her partners about her beliefs, feelings, and commitments. She followed her passion, opened New York City's first vegan shoe store, and there she met her (vegan) match.

An Unexpected Turn
Sarah W., Editor, Writer, and Writing Instructor

An editor and writer, Sarah seems to be particularly skilled at analyzing what surrounds her and picking up small but important pieces of information. By detecting what might be relevant to her life, she found veganism.

Already a vegetarian, the vegan spark lit up in Sarah at a wedding when she met a fellow attendee and noticed what she was eating. "We started talking 'cause the reception was all barbecue food . . . I just had some veggies and cheese on my plate, and she only had veggies . . . I said, 'Oh, are you vegetarian?' And she said, 'Well actually I'm vegan.'"

The two struck up a conversation and Sarah's newfound friend advised her, "just to let my conscience be my guide, and keep learning, and do what I felt was right for me . . . It wasn't pushy or anything." Soon Sarah cut the remaining animal products out of her life.

Sarah's motivations were ethical. "I've always loved animals," she explains, "and that's always been kind of in the back of my mind, how we sort of arbitrarily choose which animals that we've domesticated or have become pets . . . which animals are okay to eat and how that changes depending on where you live in the world . . ."

Sarah credits author and speaker Colleen Patrick-Goudreau as having influenced her approach to veganism—and teaching her to live with a "fully open heart, and being compassionate . . ."

When Sarah first went vegetarian, and then vegan, her then-husband was an omnivore. ". . . [H]e was fine with me cutting out meat, because we didn't eat a whole ton of meat beforehand," says Sarah. However, when she decided to go vegan, there was some apprehension at home when her husband worried that it would be difficult to find food she could eat.

Sarah stuck with what she knew was right for her, having listened to her own heart and mind, and soon her husband discovered that shopping vegan was not so difficult after all. The two continued to coexist. Occasionally they would watch a TV show or movie together that addressed animal cruelty and veganism, which would inspire them to talk about the issues. He asked Sarah questions, and she filled him in on the facts.

Then one day her husband delivered some news: "I haven't been eating any meat for the last couple of weeks . . . I'm not gonna call myself vegetarian . . . but I'm just going to be eating vegetarian for the most part . . ." Sarah says that he "came to that realization of his own sense of ethics and values," not because she was urging him in that direction.

Sarah did what was best for her, and her husband discovered that abstaining from eating animals was better for him, too. However, the two eventually went their separate ways and divorced.

"He ended up being supportive of my veganism," says Sarah about her ex-husband, "and even became vegetarian himself, but at first he was like really sort of reactionary about it, which was one of the struggles."

When Sarah began dating again, she became involved with a fellow vegan, Nathan. They are now married.

Though she didn't require that a new partner be vegan, Sarah appreciates that Nathan was living a cruelty-free lifestyle before the two became involved with each other. "It's night and day," she says, "not only being with someone who is generally supportive and respectful of my opinions and lifestyle, but someone who's also on their own embraced being vegan."

There are qualities that Sarah believes are essential to herself and Nathan, that brought them both to veganism, and connect them to each other: "I think both of us are in a way dreamers and idealists," she says, "doing something to make the world a better place. And I think that sort of open-heartedness, open-mindedness, compassion, and empathy is for sure what drew me to him."

The two have much in common in addition to veganism. They share a passion for writing. "We love good stories, good characters," says Sarah, and they like playing video games together. Sarah has also enjoyed combining their companion animals into one home.

Following her divorce, Sarah didn't set out to partner with a vegan; in fact, she told Nathan that if he ever returned to being an omnivore, she wouldn't be upset. However, by listening to her conscience, and following her heart to someone she connected with, she landed in a happy home with another vegan, two dogs, and a cat.

Vegan Love Rises Above the Differences
Jasmin Singer, Cohost of the Our Hen House Podcast and Author

Fierce female Jasmin Singer has been a vegan and very active animal activist for more than a decade. She is a cofounder of the animal rights nonprofit media hub *Our Hen House* and an accomplished writer who authored the memoir *Always Too Much and Never Enough*.

Jasmin has always made it a general rule to be totally and unapologetically open and honest about her veganism with everyone she meets from the get-go. "It's impossible to know anything about me and not know I'm vegan. It's related to my profession, and my tattoos. So I don't think there's much of a guessing game there . . ."

What has worked for Jasmin in every other area of her life has historically worked for her in the romantic realm. Jasmin has found dating success in being completely up-front from day one. Her joyously confrontational style, from her jet-black hair to her colorful tattoos, matches her strong and bold voice for the animals. By letting who she really is rise and shine, she has not only found veganism, but her career, friends, and romantic partners.

Jasmin has dated a number of non-vegans who eventually moved toward a plant-based diet. "When you have that kind of an intimate relationship with someone, their defenses tend to be down a bit, which is a perfect time to talk to them about the many reasons you are vegan." When she began dating as a vegan, Jasmin didn't exclude omnivores from the dating pool; however, she did have some guidelines. "I was always adamant that the person be open to changing and becoming vegan," she explains. It was a rule that she had taken time to consider carefully, looking inside herself and acknowledging her feelings. Jasmin realized that indeed, this was a prerequisite—she could not be happy in a relationship with someone who would not consider veganism.

After years of exploring relationships with vegan-curious omnivores, Jasmin reached a turning point when she realized it was important to her to be only with another vegan. "I became what I guess you'd call a vegan-sexual," she says.

"Dating only vegans was always my ideal situation, but it didn't always work out that way. So I moved to only dating people who were extremely open to becoming vegan (that is, if the vegans were all taken)," says Jasmin. "It was such a breath of fresh air when I finally connected with a vegan woman who was also an animal activist, like me. In addition to our deep connection and shared worldview, the fact she was so heavily enmeshed in the world of animal rights, and such a longtime vegan, was something I craved in a partner. It was so important to me, after having dated so many non-vegans, that my partner know the ropes.

"Alongside another vegan, I can do everything from cry when the enormity of the reality of animal suffering gets the better of me; to share in the delight of an amazing new vegan restaurant or product; to—and perhaps this is the best piece—not even need to discuss anything about my veganism, because it's just accepted, never questioned. My veganism is the best part of me, and sharing that with a partner makes the connection that much deeper and stronger."

Says Jasmin, "If you can handle dating a non-vegan—with the secret (or not so secret) intent to convert them—go for it. I think there is a moral argument in favor of each of us dating our fair share of non-vegans, and converting them, before becoming vegansexuals. . . . But if that's not an option for you, then I totally get that. There is nothing greater than sharing your life with someone who truly gets it and gets you, no questions asked. Since the vegan dating pool is indeed a relatively small one, you might want to reassess your other prerequisites. Is it age? Gender? Something else? Even if someone appears to be an unlikely match for you, I suggest keeping your mind and heart open. You may see eye to eye on important issues that trump the other ones."

A Vegan Is Born
Robyn Lazara, Birth and Postpartum Doula Care, Childbirth Educator

Robyn Lazara and her husband, Bryan, are both vegan in the interest of saving animals from suffering. Throughout the years, Robyn has shifted from being a single omnivore employed on Wall Street to a married mother working as a doula and childbirth educator. With her deep-rooted maternal instincts and soulful demeanor, it's hard to imagine her positioned behind a desk in the Financial District, but that's exactly where she was when she found veganism.

In 2005, one of Robyn's friends at her Wall Street office approached her about taking a trip to a vegetarian spa (which was actually mostly vegan except for the occasional appearance of casein—a protein present in milk). Explains Robyn, "There were always these ridiculous competitions going on in the workplace that I didn't choose to take part in, but a very close friend of mine was doing this 'Biggest Loser' competition with the guys on the trading floor, and she really wanted to get a leg up on all of them." The friend decided that going to the spa was a great way to lose weight to get ahead in the competition, and she invited Robyn. Without giving it much thought, Robyn agreed to go. She went on a whim, and it changed her life.

Beginning on January 1, 2006, the pair spent a week at the Florida spa—eating (mostly) vegan, exercising, and attending health lectures. Robyn returned to freezing cold New York City feeling great and committed to a healthy lifestyle. She ate mostly vegetarian during the months following the trip and says, "I guess just the practice of eating this way opened my heart and mind to what was going on with the animals, because not too long afterwards I started finding out about factory farming and what the animals go through . . . I became a staunchly ethical vegan." By dramatically reducing the suffering in her diet, Robyn was able to connect with the animals and soon found herself in a place of cutting out more of the cruelty. Robyn also became an activist, speaking out for animals who cannot speak for themselves.

Robyn came to be vegan by doing what was best for the animals she shares the planet with. But some of those in her life didn't embrace the change: "Friends that I had at the time stopped inviting me to things, and one of them really got on this tangent about how socially limiting it was to be vegan, which I find hilarious now that I have this huge wide circle of vegan friends." Robyn didn't let detractors sway her, and her social life flourished with many new friends who shared her principles and lifestyle. She even began hosting vegan "meetups"—gatherings usually held at vegan and vegetarian restaurants in New York City.

At one such meetup, Robyn first encountered the man who would become her husband. Bryan, a vegan, and Robyn had mutual friends but didn't meet until he sat directly across from her at an event she had organized at a Brooklyn café. Robyn says of Bryan, "we were friends for two years, and then started dating . . . he had had feelings for me and I didn't realize it . . ." They have been together ever since, and married in 2011.

Though Robyn did date some non-vegans before becoming involved with Bryan, when it came to a long-term relationship and marriage, she chose a vegan partner. Says Robyn of having a cruelty-free mate: "Well it's really just incredible . . . There's no debate, we eat vegan food together . . . our son eats vegan food . . . It's part of the foundation of our relationship . . . So much of being in a relationship is having shared values and beliefs, and this is really a core one."

Robyn does point out that their shared veganism is not the only thing holding her and Bryan together. "We enjoy each other's company," she says. "We really like being around and with each other." She adds, "He's an incredibly endearing person, incredibly sweet and generous and kind-hearted."

Having the core belief of veganism in common with her husband is important to Robyn: "It's a really reassuring thing to have whether or not you're planning to have children—just to have shared ethics," she says. "I could never end up paired with somebody who's homophobic or racist . . . speciesism is pretty profound . . ." Robyn does not want to share a home with someone who is prejudiced against non-human animals as much as she would not want to be with someone who puts down others based on their race or sexual orientation.

An Activist Couple Is a Happy Couple
Kara Davis, Animal Advocate and Publishing Professional

Cat moms to six furry little ones at home, and looking after a feral colony of three, Kara and Korn show their love for animals in the daily care of their four-legged companions, through their activism, and with their shared vegan lifestyle. Now living in Beacon, New York, the two met because of their mutual engagement in queer and anti-police brutality causes in New York City. Although for Kara animal rights went hand in hand with her other activism, she found that many within the social justice activist community did not feel the same way and frowned upon animal causes. She says that one of the things she and Korn initially liked about each other was their mutual involvement with and concern for animals—and that they were both vegetarian.

Kara has been vegan twice. She originally cut out animal products in the eighties, but after a cross-country move, found herself feeling isolated. Says Kara, "I was not only vegan, I was heavily involved in animal rights activism when I moved to the East Coast. I didn't know anybody and eventually was depressed, and it seemed much harder . . ." Kara didn't become an omnivore, but vegetarian, more out of feeling alone than as a conscious decision.

"It was always there, was always percolating," says Kara about her and Korn's decision to go vegan together. ". . . I missed having a commitment to veganism and she was willing to try it."

Korn and Kara came to veganism by way of the very interest that had introduced the pair in the first place—their activism. The two signed up for an activist training camp in Florida, and when offered the option of having vegan meals while there, they decided to try it for the three-week trip.

While at the training camp, debate erupted when two attendees voiced upset at the camp's solely vegetarian and vegan food offerings. The protesting parties argued that vegetarianism was racist and didn't take their own cultural lives into account. On the one hand, says Kara, "Culture and entire *cultures* that are being wiped out . . . are something to fight to keep alive. But *culture* also describes a living, evolving thing that demands consideration and reconsideration and analysis, like art." She continues, "Slavery and racism and harsh border controls are a part of my white United States southwestern culture, as are big guns and domestic violence and severe alcoholism. Animal eating is a part of *most* cultures, but that doesn't mean it has to be swallowed as a positive part, or that it can't change."

"[T]he camp basically shut down," says Kara, "and it all became a discussion of racism and vegetarianism." Originally from Brazil, Korn was picked out during the debate as an example of a Latina immigrant who cared about vegetarianism. "My girlfriend is from the northeast of Brazil," says Kara. "Meat-eating was a gigantic part of any meal or celebration [there]. But that's changing for a lot of people as they become concerned about their health, the disappearance of the rain forest, the sale of the country's valuable western land to United States beef industries, and the theft of land from native groups. Being vegetarian does not make someone less Brazilian, or of any place or culture."

Being used as an example in this situation was an awkward and frustrating role for Korn, who already struggles with accusations of "over-assimilation" because of being queer and no longer having an accent. Says Kara, "Discussions about labor abuse and environmental racism (in animal production), as well as feminist opposition to dairy and egg production, brought to the forefront all the reasons that I've been vegan and interested in veganism. The discourse also brought up for Korn how much she cared about animals and what she wanted to do for them, so that was it. We went home and were vegan forever after."

Having open conversations while becoming vegan together helped Kara and Korn clarify their opinions and manage the actions they took in response to their new lifestyle. "[W]e had discussions about whether we should get rid of clothes or things that we already had, but because we were pretty broke, we didn't. We had conversations about how . . . [veganism is] about causing the least pain possible, not about purity . . ."

In becoming vegan again, Kara had the opposite experience of the isolation she found when she'd arrived on the East Coast. The shift reignited her engagement in animal activism, and she met many like-minded people.

Kara advises vegan women to "make sure you have other people concerned with this stuff in your life, and it doesn't have to be the person you're dating." Connecting with other vegans can make a huge difference for us when it comes to making a difference for animals. For those of us who are vegan, it can feel very basic to our identity, a core value. In a world where one's commitment to veganism is often challenged by outspoken omnivores, meat-slinging restaurants, and articles in news outlets, it can be very helpful to have the emotional reinforcement of others in your life who share this worldview.

How to Meet a Vegan: They Don't Grow on Trees

Although vegans are plant-based, we don't grow on trees. However, we are many in numbers. Here are some places where you might meet cruelty-free partners.

Farm Animal Sanctuaries

With the growing vegan movement, an increasing number of farm animal sanctuaries are establishing themselves across the United States and internationally. Many of these host events, such as Farm Sanctuary's annual Hoe Downs, or cooking classes 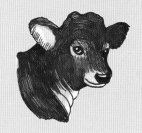 at Catskill Animal Sanctuary, which attract vegans from near and far.

Vegan Meetups

According to the *Meetup* website, there are nearly 1,500 "Vegan Meetups" around the globe, in cities ranging from Singapore to

Chicago. These groups organize meetings of their members that range from meals at vegan-friendly restaurants to activist excursions. With that many groups, you are bound to meet someone up to your dating standards.

Book Signings

You may have noticed an abundance of books being published on vegan issues. Looking for a bookish type? A signing at a local shop may be the perfect place to find one. Make sure to raise your hand and ask a question during the Q&A to draw attention to yourself and your informed interest in the topic. Can't find one in your area? Organize one!

Veg Fests

Vegan and vegetarian festivals are held regularly throughout North America, collecting those interested in plant-based living to peruse booths with cruelty-free products, sit in on fascinating lectures, and sometimes learn to cook a vegan dish or two. Opportunities to meet fellow vegans are plenty. You can always use the old trick of "accidentally" knocking someone's pamphlets out of their hands and then helping to pick them up.

Activism

For many of us, going vegan and attending activist activities go hand in hand. When I first went vegetarian, I went to many meetings for an anti-foie gras campaign, at which I found myself surrounded by like-minded people.

There's nothing quite like the energy of a protest, and they provide a great opportunity to see others' passion (or find out you don't see eye to eye with someone). Protests bring people's core beliefs to the fore and are a great scenario to find out if you connect with a fellow activist.

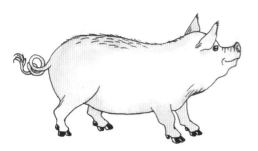

CHAPTER 6

There's a Place For Us: Vegan-Friendly Date Destinations

Some date destinations are clearly vegan-unfriendly. Circuses with animal performers, fishing excursions, and zoos—which deny animals their freedom—would obviously not be good options. Some gray areas also exist when it comes to cruelty-free date destinations. A day at the museum sounds lovely, but will you be able to eat at the restaurant? Dates are meant to be fun, for both people. If we make suggestions, ask questions, and do research when necessary, we can help ensure that our ethics won't be challenged.

Painting the Town Vegan

This past Fourth of July weekend, I went on one of my favorite dates ever with my partner. We drove to Woodstock Farm Sanctuary for a "jamboree," where we spent time with rescued animals who live there and indulged in delicious vegan food. Finding a spot with friends at a picnic table, we lounged in the shade, chatting about our favorite bands from the eighties, books, and a new vegan TV show. My boyfriend, the animals, friends, and delicious vegan food—who could ask for anything more?

Spending time at a farm animal sanctuary, whether for a tour, an event, or an overnight stay, could possibly be the perfect date for any vegan. But what if that vegan has an omnivore partner? Women who I spoke to for this book told me that the omnivores in their lives enjoyed their time at these peaceful shelters for rescued animals, too. In one case, a formerly omnivorous husband left the sanctuary a new vegan.

I love the time I spend with my partner at farm animal sanctuaries, but I probably wouldn't have suggested one for our first date. I think of first dates as setting the stage to get to know each other, and for a non-vegan, a first date at a sanctuary could feel like their love interest is trying to teach them a lesson.

For first dates, I usually opted for more local locales. I found that when I let someone know about my compassionate lifestyle, they usually took time to figure out a place for our date that would suit both of us. This signaled to me that they were thoughtful, empathetic humans who took into consideration my love of animals. One of the greatest lessons I learned in dating was that expressing my needs as a vegan (in a kind way) was a very good thing, and if a person didn't respect what I needed to feel comfortable, he wasn't a good partner for me.

When I dove back into dating following my recovery from cancer, I worried that telling a potential partner I was vegan would make me seem "high maintenance," but I learned that being a confident, happy vegan actually made me more desirable to many. I realized that any person who did not think veganism was a positive, admirable, respectable way of living was not someone who I wanted to be with.

I learned that the men who I respected and admired most also respected and admired my veganism. On our first date, my boyfriend came out to Brooklyn (an hour and a half trip from his home) to dine with me at a vegan restaurant. He didn't see it as an inconvenience, but seemed happy to accommodate me.

A very accomplished and eligible (omnivore) male friend of mine always requests we go to a plant-based restaurant when I meet him for lunch. I've learned that going to a vegan restaurant doesn't have to translate to a compromise for an omnivore, and some of the most talented, intelligent, single non-vegans I know are excited to eat delicious, creatively prepared cruelty-free foods.

As a vegan, I would certainly want to avoid some destinations for dates. I would never want to go to a circus with animals, a zoo, or any other venue where living beings are held captive to be used as entertainment. I would also want to avoid any restaurant that doesn't offer appealing vegan options.

There are plenty of great places for vegan dates. I've visited many museums in cities including Vienna and Montreal with my boyfriend, that didn't compromise my veganism. Wandering around these magnificent institutions, we learned more about each other's tastes and loves, likes and dislikes. In Berlin, we enjoyed spending hours on a stormy day gazing at the massive pieces adorning a museum's walls.

Often we want to be outside. My boyfriend is an avid hiker and though I was born and raised in a city, I too have a great love of the outdoors. We both like long walks in the woods, a wonderful way to experience nature that is very vegan-friendly. Sometimes we talk about the beauty unfolding around us, and sometimes we are quiet as we take it in. Occasionally we have the opportunity to see animals in their natural environment or hear their noises in the distance. Last night we strolled along the edge of the Hudson River, stepping on the rocky beach. We saw a family of ducks as they swam in the water, the ducklings running to shore when the waves began to get rough, mama close behind.

When we're feeling truly adventurous, my partner and I go camping. These trips require more planning than most of our other dates, but we find that the preparation brings us together. We enjoy creating a list of what we need, visiting the supply store, and planning our meals as a couple. Camping may present some stressful situations (pouring rain, a fire that won't start), and working through those challenges can make us closer—but I might not pick such an involved outing as the setting for a first or second date.

Of course, as much as I enjoy dates with my boyfriend, whether we go to a fine vegan restaurant or casual takeout place, visit a museum or go on a camping trip, there will always be things I like to do that he doesn't. I love to lounge in front of the TV with a cup of coffee and he would much rather practice playing guitar. I enjoy book launch parties and he'd rather stay at home.

Though I go on many fun, exciting, and sometimes adventurous dates with my partner, I still go on dates with myself. Inevitably there will be activities I enjoy that he doesn't. That's okay. I can still do those things. It doesn't mean I love him (or that he'll love me) any less. There are plenty of great vegan dates to share with my boyfriend, and there are some I enjoy on my own.

Great Places For Vegans, Date Destinations to Avoid, and Figuring Out the In-Between

Being vegan doesn't mean giving up great options for dates. Who would want an outing with someone we are interested in to involve cruelty? Dating is all about connecting with another person, so why would we want to see an animal hurt in the process?

There are plenty of ways to spend a date that don't involve cruelty to animals, though there are some scenarios you may want to avoid.

For instance, if a date suggests going to a zoo or aquarium, where animals are held against their will, the moment to speak up is now. I try not to criticize the other person when voicing my veganism, yet offer a sound explanation for why I'm opting out of an activity. A good response to a zoo invitation might be, "I don't like seeing animals in cages, but it would be nice to be outdoors. Why don't we go to the park instead?" In this way, you can lightly broach the subject of why you stay away from zoos, but build on a positive aspect of your date's idea. Once you know this person a little better, perhaps you can have a more in-depth conversation with them about the issues. You can stand strong in your vegan shoes without lashing out at someone else. No one wants to feel judged by the person they are interested in. And remember, most of us were not born vegan and had to learn these lessons for ourselves. Think about how you would want someone to have treated you when you were not yet vegan.

If you pause for a moment when someone suggests a date that offends your ethics, and consider what it is they perceive as fun, you may be able to come up with a great vegan alternative. Say a date or partner wants to go fishing—why not suggest apple-picking instead? Nobody gets hurt! Fishing may be a tradition in your partner's family, but perhaps what they really enjoy about it is being outside and harvesting food—an activity that is easily veganized.

Restaurants

Many people think of a fine restaurant as an ideal destination for a date. Say an omnivore offers to take you to their favorite steak house for your first meeting, but you find out they serve no vegan options. It isn't likely that your date picked that place because of the animal cruelty involved. What does that restaurant have to offer that may be drawing your date to it? Lovely ambience, outdoor seating, creatively prepared food? Simply think of what the vegan equivalent might be. No fancy vegan restaurants in your area? There are probably some elegant establishments that offer delicious plant-based dishes. A gentle explanation such as, "I don't eat animal products," followed by a suggestion that reflects the positive aspects of your date's idea should do the trick: "I know another restaurant I think you'll like that also has a lovely vibe but with great vegan options." If a date isn't willing to be flexible to suit your needs, is he or she really a person you want to be involved with?

Movies

Movies can be great for dates, as long as you can find a film you both want to see. A movie theater offers both an opportunity to enjoy an experience together and vegan snacks aplenty. If you're feeling confused at the snack bar, you can look at the Quick Guide in chapter 7, which lists which cinema treats are vegan.

Live Music

Similar to movies, seeing live music is a great vegan-friendly way to spend a first date. While you're deciding which concert to go to, you may learn more about the other person's taste. Live music can be a physical experience, often with dancing and the *thump thump thump* of the bass. If you are interested in someone but wary of getting too intimate too quickly, seeing a band play is a way to share a physical experience without hopping into bed with them right away.

Museums and Historical Sites

Museums and historical destinations can offer wonderful settings to take in great artworks and pieces of history with someone whose company you enjoy. However, if you plan to eat at a museum or historical site restaurant, you might want to call ahead. As convenient as it may be to have lunch while you're there, you'll want to be sure there's something vegan available. If not, you can suggest a place close by to lunch after you've taken in all of the beauty and history.

Many historical sites have outdoor areas that are great for picnicking. Check the restrictions in advance, and if outdoor eating is allowed, why not pack a delicious vegan meal for two?

The Great Outdoors

Having spent most of my life in the city, I don't have too much experience with the great outdoors, but I love it. In the few years I've been with my nature-loving partner, I've had the opportunity to go on many hikes, walks, and a few campouts. Hiking and camping are wonderful ways of communing with nature and getting to know the person you are with. Surprisingly, although being in nature allows us to see animals living in their true homes, parks and campsites can be somewhat vegan unfriendly, as many people grill meat while there.

My boyfriend, who has been vegan since we began dating, and vegetarian for many years before that, has a very sensitive sense of smell. He abhors the scent of cooking meat. When we go to Brooklyn's Prospect Park for walks (one of our favorite dates), we are quick to pass by the designated barbecue areas. We run into the same challenge when we go camping. Smoke wafting over from another campsite can pose a real challenge for us. So we try to plan in advance. Strolling in the park, and when camping, we try to stay away from stinky smoke by steering clear of grilling areas. Some campsites will allow more distance between tents than others, decreasing the chance that you will get a whiff of someone else's cooking. This space is something you may want to consider when planning your trip.

There's no reason to refrain from enjoying beautiful parks and campsites, but you might want to do so mindfully.

Friends and Family

If you continue to date someone, at some point you will probably meet their friends and family. This often takes place at a party or other large gathering where you may not be in control of the menu. Going with a new partner to meet those they hold near and dear can be stressful to begin with, let alone worrying about what you will eat. Some of us are concerned that claiming our veganism and explaining our needs may leave a bad impression. But of course there is nothing bad about being vegan. Find a quiet time to speak to your partner about your concerns and they may offer to ask their friends or family about vegan options. If they're not willing, or there is no cruelty-free food on the menu, you can offer to bring a great vegan dish for everyone to enjoy. What better way of introducing yourself than to offer fantastic plant-based food that the whole party can indulge in?

Trips Abroad

Who doesn't love a destination date? Haven't we all dreamed of being whisked away to someplace special for the weekend? There's no reason we can't have this ultimate romantic experience with our lover while staying true to our vegan selves. For international getaways, airlines offer vegan meals, just be sure to call in advance to reserve yours. Though some locales are more vegan-friendly than others, I have never found a destination devoid of vegan food options. Even in St. Martin, which offers predominantly French (often meat and dairy heavy) cuisine, my boyfriend and I discovered the Freedom Fighters Ital Shack, which serves up divine all-vegan food. In fact, some of my favorite meals have been the ones my partner and I have had at little-known eateries in foreign cities. Often we use the *Happy Cow* website or cell phone "app" to sort out which restaurants have vegan options. Websites can be great tools, but they aren't necessary to find vegan food. When we were deep in the German countryside without a *Happy Cow* listing to be found, we made our way to a Chinese restaurant and found a few items to order. I can't think of a cuisine that doesn't use plants. Even if you are someplace that seems vegan-unfriendly, a gentle request for a meal that suits your specifications should result in something you can dine on.

Sharing the Vegan Love

If you're involved with a fellow vegan, you may already have been making the rounds as a couple to animal sanctuaries, vegan book events, and films addressing the issues. If you are dating an omnivore you may have been sticking with more neutral territory such as movies and concerts. Once there is a level of trust, and an omnivore partner knows they're not being judged, you might want to take your dates to a new vegan level.

Like author JL Fields (who we'll meet in chapter 8), many people believe that non-vegans simply aren't vegans yet, and that we all may have our moment of realizing we want to cut the cruelty out of our lives. To have that moment, however, many omnivores need to be in a place where they can learn, whether it's at a talk, a film screening, or a sanctuary. For an omnivore who isn't feeling too defensive, vegan events such as panel discussions and film showings can be fantastic date destinations. We don't want our partners to feel that they're going to these events against their will, though. If we are enthusiastic and extend a friendly invitation, the omnivores in our lives may just follow their hearts to join us at a vegan event.

Farm animal sanctuaries can be exceptionally great settings for omnivores to start down a vegan path. Many people have been inspired to cut out the cruelty after visiting one of these peaceful places and meeting cows, pigs, goats, sheep, turkeys, and chickens in person. If your partner is expressing curiosity about your compassionate choices, why not suggest a trip to meet animals who have been rescued from the food industry?

I Want to Take You Higher:
Planning a Vegan-Friendly Date

At their best, dates give us the opportunity to connect with another person while experiencing something fun, adventurous, or even educational together. When they go well, we may come away from the date feeling lighthearted and joyful. Of course, what really makes time together great is the connection you share with your partner, but here are some vegan-friendly date ideas that may help you achieve that high.

Roller Skating—Whether you're a true beginner or an expert, roller skating together can be a great way to let down your guard and simply have fun. The music, lights, and the joy of spinning around the floor make this much more than just exercise.

To Veganize: Most roller skates are leather. You can call ahead to find out whether a rink's skates are vegan. If they're not, you can easily purchase cruelty-free versions online.

A Botanical Garden—Who doesn't love a stroll among beautiful flowers? Many cities have delightful botanical gardens with long paths through fields of blooms and meticulously manicured lawns.

To Veganize: Call ahead to check if the snack bar or restaurant offers vegan options for your lunch. If not, find out the garden's picnic policy. What could be more romantic than spreading out and dining al fresco, surrounded by flowers?

On the Water—Many of us are not too far from a body of water, whether it's a lake, a river, or an ocean. Water offers plenty of activities to pick from, which are especially inviting on a hot summer day. Kayaking on a river, splashing in a country watering hole, or touring a city on a riverboat—being on the water can offer a wonderful otherworldly experience.

To Veganize: If you're going to be on a boat for a meal, you'll want to call ahead to confirm there are vegan options. When my boyfriend and I floated through Berlin on a riverboat, french fries were available but nothing else that fit the vegan bill. It's easy to pack something portable to eat if you know in advance that you'll need it.

Dinner and a Movie—A time-tested tradition, dinner and a movie can be a great way to spend an evening with a new love or committed partner. This classic combination can be budget-friendly (without sacrificing the fun-factor), or made more extravagant by dining at an elegant restaurant.

To Veganize: If you're meeting someone who is not familiar with your compassionate lifestyle, you can gently fill them in and suggest a vegan-friendly restaurant that they may also enjoy. Once at the movies, dig in if you'd like to. There are plenty of vegan treats for sale in most theaters. (See Quick Guide: Vegan/Not Vegan Movie Theater Treats in chapter 7.)

A Home-Cooked Evening—Once you've established a person you are dating isn't a danger, why not invite them over? This is a great way to share your world with them. You can sit on the couch together, sipping drinks by candlelight, and have a relaxed meal with your favorite music in the background. You might even want to pull out a board game.

To Veganize: Since it's your home, you don't need to worry about any items or dinner ingredients not being vegan. However, your guest may want to contribute something to the evening such as dessert or a bottle of wine. A gentle reminder that you keep a vegan home and to please only bring cruelty-free items should do the trick.

CHAPTER 7

Sipping, Supping, and Munching Vegan on Dates: Cruelty-Free Food and Booze

Dining out and drinking are often the focal points of dates. This makes a lot of sense since most of us eat and drink multiple times each day. Many people won't think twice before inviting you to dinner or coffee at their favorite spot. But that place may not be vegan-friendly. Arriving at a restaurant, bar, or café prepared can save you the worry of not knowing what items are cruelty-free.

Eat, Drink, and Be Wary

As a vegan, I am always disappointed when I order a dish in a restaurant and discover upon its arrival that it contains animal products. The good news is that when we ask the right questions, most of the time we can prevent this from happening.

If one's date is very vegan-friendly, that person may want to join you at a plant-based restaurant. Many non-vegans embrace the opportunity to try a delicious cruelty-free meal. In that case, you're safe since everything on the menu will be animal-free.

However, if you land at a non-vegan restaurant, there's no guarantee that any menu offerings will be free from animal products. Though this may require educating yourself about the food available and could mean requesting dishes not listed, it can also be an opportunity to serve as a vegan ambassador.

Many of us have been taught that asking for what we need makes us "high maintenance" or "difficult." There is a modern (and old) myth that by speaking up about what we require, we are making life hard for others. The truth is that whenever I have spoken up for myself in regard to my veganism, the response has generally been positive and helpful. I can honestly say that no one has ever rolled their eyes at me, become hostile, or debated with me when I've inquired as to whether a dish is vegan.

In fact, time and again I have received encouraging, positive responses from waiters and waitresses in restaurants, and sometimes even questions about veganism, opening up an opportunity to educate someone else about the benefits of a plant-based diet. One time, dining in an Indian restaurant, my partner and I asked a waiter if dairy ghee was used in the dishes. Ghee (a common ingredient in Indian food) is typically derived from butter, though vegetable ghee is also available. The waiter inquired why we abstain from dairy products, and so we shared our ethical reasons. He listened to us and then smiled, deeming us "saints," and commending us on our lifestyle. My boyfriend and I may not be saints, but labeling us as such is a far cry from antagonism. Clearly this person did not find us high maintenance or difficult.

If you are in a restaurant and one of the establishment's staff asks you a question about your vegan requirements, this presents you with a great opportunity to represent vegans in a positive way. You may not want to read a prepared speech, but if you are kind and respectful, speaking to that person how you would want to be spoken to in your omnivore days (since most of us were formerly omnivores), you can be a great ambassador. Every time a person asks us a question about our compassionate lifestyle, we have the opportunity to dispel the image of the angry vegan. Though people have various reasons for being omnivores, many simply haven't been exposed to basic information about the cruelties of farming. Any time you speak about your veganism with an omnivore, you may be shining a light on something they are in the dark about. By being kind when we speak to others, we can invite people in, rather than making them feel badly for their own choices.

I love going to restaurants. Admittedly, my boyfriend and I will often dine out multiple times in a week. I believe in the benefits of eating at home, too, but I enjoy the experience of going to another space, taking in an ambience someone else has created, and indulging in food that I probably could not have prepared myself.

Through the years, I've been to many wonderful vegan restaurants. We met the married owners of three of New York City's finest vegan establishments, the Candle restaurants, in chapter 5. My boyfriend and I have eaten at Candle 79 (one of the three) on numerous special occasions. Another of my favorites is the Loving Hut chain of vegan restaurants, which I've eaten at in cities around the world including Hanoi, Vienna, and San Francisco.

However, my boyfriend and I often dine in non-vegan establishments. We love Thai, Indian, Mediterranean, and Chinese food and frequently eat these cuisines, usually in restaurants that are not entirely plant-based. We just know to ask some very specific questions when we go to a restaurant for the first time.

When eating Thai food, there are two ingredients in particular that I generally ask about: fish sauce and egg. A favorite Thai dish for many is pad thai. Though regularly served with these non-vegan ingredients, most restaurants can accommodate a plant-based diet by leaving them out of their recipe. Though some servers will know what "vegan" means, I generally take the approach of explaining that I don't eat any animal products, mentioning some examples. Veganism is growing, and chances are your server has encountered a vegan before, but if not, this is a great opportunity to gently educate them while you are making sure that your meal is cruelty-free.

My boyfriend and I also frequent a local Chinese restaurant. Though the restaurant has an extensive selection of vegetable dishes, whether they are vegan isn't indicated on the menu. When we order a dish there, we confirm that the broths used are vegetable-derived and ask about other animal products. Then we enjoy a great meal.

Whether I'm traveling or at home, I often go to Mediterranean restaurants. Though some of the dishes in most of these restaurants are meat-based, there are often many vegan-friendly ones. Some of my favorites are falafel (chickpea-based patties), baba ghanoush (a dip-like dish made of roasted eggplant), and beet salad. I'm getting hungry just thinking about all of that great food. So just because 100 percent of the menu at my favorite Mediterranean spot isn't plant-based, doesn't mean I won't eat well. However, if I go to a new restaurant, I ask a few questions. One restaurant I've been to adds non-vegan mayonnaise to their baba ghanoush and hummus, traditionally vegan dishes.

Another one of my favorite cuisines is Japanese. However, unless the restaurant is all-vegan, there's a chance that eel sauce or another animal ingredients, such as bonito flakes (made of fish) may be used. If you take a moment to ask a friendly question, you should be able to find out.

I've learned not to take anything for granted when I go to a restaurant for the first time and consider asking a few questions to be routine. If something isn't vegan as prepared, often the animal ingredients can be left out.

Of course there are different ways to ask a question. If we are gentle, kind, and respectful when speaking with the staff at restaurants, we are not only good ambassadors for veganism, but we may impress our dates.

If you've asked all of the questions (are those vegetables cooked in butter? Is there cheese in that salad? Can you leave off the eel sauce?) and can't seem to find a vegan dish, most eateries can provide steamed vegetables and rice or another combination of vegan ingredients. Though no vegan option may be listed, most restaurants are able to prepare a plant-based meal upon request.

Does the demon that warns you not to be high maintenance raise its head when you think about asking these questions on a date? One of the greatest lessons I've learned is to always be true to myself, even if I am imperfect at it. Though these fears may lurk in the back of our heads, in my experience, the people who I respect the most also respect me for voicing my needs. If someone doesn't regard the expression of my truth as a positive thing, then this is probably not a person I want to be around. That doesn't mean that I'm antagonistic toward people who don't support me, but if someone were to make me feel uncomfortable for speaking up for myself and the animals, I would be inclined to separate from that person. A person who eats meat doesn't express their truth by disparaging a vegan.

Why would you want to be around someone who denied you a beautiful part of yourself?

Navigating Cafés, Bars, and Snacks

The truth is that vegan food is not hard to find. For a moment, think about how many plant-based ingredients there are—myriad vegetables; fruits from apples to kiwis; grains like oats, rice, and millet; nuts including everything from almonds to walnuts to cashews; seeds from pumpkins and sunflowers. Not to mention a vast variety of vegan meats and cheeses. Now think about what ingredients aren't vegan: meat, dairy, eggs, honey, etc. There are so many plant-based foods that we are really not denying ourselves much when we cut out the non-vegan ingredients. If we miss the taste of animal foods, there is usually a vegan replacement for what we're excluding. Many plant-based meats nearly exactly replicate the taste of the animal-derived originals. I've eaten delicious vegan yogurt made from almond milk and sipped tea sweetened with agave, a cruelty-free syrup that easily takes the place of honey.

Given the foods that the earth offers us, it's easy to eat an entirely plant-based diet. What can be challenging is eating vegan when the food is prepared by someone else, whether we're eating in a café or purchasing a snack in a store. It may be surprising to some who enjoy drinking in bars to learn that many beers and wines are also not vegan. However, with some proper preparation, all of these scenarios are easy to navigate.

Cafés

I love going to cafés on dates. They are cute but casual, often quite cozy, and one can simply sip a drink or opt-in for food. I also like that they generally offer an amount of intimacy, but are public so that I feel I am in a safe place when just getting to know someone. It was in a delightful café in Rosendale, New York, that my boyfriend asked me why I was vegan, and then decided to go vegan himself.

Many cafés offer clearly labeled vegan dishes on their menus. For those that don't, I would suggest doing some research ahead of time to find out what you'll be able to eat (and drink). A quick phone call will usually give you the clarity you need, but if you're stopping somewhere spontaneously, you should still be able to find something to order.

If you're planning to drink tea or coffee with milk, you'll want to ask if the café offers soy, almond, or another non-dairy milk option.

Let's say you'd like to eat on your café date and there are no dishes on the menu that are marked vegan. Your next step might be asking the server which options don't contain animal products. If that person tells you that they don't know, or that nothing is vegan, you're still not out of luck. Many salads and sandwiches that aren't plant-based can be made vegan. The server should be able to let you know if the café's bread contains any animal products (such as eggs, milk, or whey). If they have vegan bread, most cafés can easily assemble an avocado, lettuce, and tomato sandwich. Yum! You'll probably want to skip the margarine in cafés, as many brands contain casein (a protein derived from milk).

If the sandwiches aren't an option, the salads might be. Perhaps the only non-vegan ingredient in a café's salads is some feta or blue cheese. Simply ask if the cheese can be left off. Just be sure to check that there's no honey or (non-vegan) mayonnaise in the dressing. Remember, you know what qualifies as animal products, but everyone may not. In securing a vegan meal, the person serving you may find it helpful to be told specific examples of foods that you don't eat: honey, milk, mayonnaise. These examples may seem obvious to you, but veganism can feel like a tricky language to learn for those who are unfamiliar with it. Are you interested in a restaurant's fall vegetables platter? You can nicely ask if butter is an ingredient.

Again, ordering food in a non-vegan café is a great opportunity to be an ambassador for all vegans. If we treat people we are explaining our veganism to with respect and kindness, they may be interested in being more helpful to other vegans. If we are condescending or antagonistic, it may lead someone to dread serving a vegan again. We have a choice in how we represent ourselves to others, and don't we want everyone to love vegans?

Being vegan can require some extra work, sometimes finding food takes more effort than we may have invested as omnivores, but the rewards are immense. For me, feeling happier, healthier, and knowing I am preventing cruelty to animals is worth every bit of energy I put into living vegan.

Bars

Bars are a classic date locale. My writing professor in college likened them to theaters, with stages set for whatever the night might bring. Many of us will opt not to drink alcohol on dates, for various reasons, but those of us who do may be surprised to learn that some seemingly plant-based drinks, including various wines and beers, are made with animal products.

Sarah Gross, who we met in chapter 4, is cofounder of the Better Booze Festival, which showcases vegan alcoholic beverages. She explains, "People just assume that alcoholic drinks are naturally vegan. But sometimes distillers use fish bladders (called isinglass) or egg whites during the filtering phase of their concoctions. And those non-vegan elements are *not* required to appear on the ingredients list (in the United States, anyway)."

Though we may think of drinks like beer and wine as plant-based, they may not be completely vegan. With a little research, we can be sure not to sip someone else's suffering.

Sarah explains that mead, another alcoholic drink, is created with honey and water, so it is also not vegan. She adds, "If there's an overly cute animal name on a cocktail, chances are it does contain that animal. For example, the Duck Duck Duck contains deviled duck heart, and the Bay of Pigs is a rum and orange drink garnished with bacon."

Though there are some alcoholic drinks that are not cruelty-free, there is a wide selection of animal-friendly options. Finding out the vegan status of your favorite beverages in advance of your date should provide you with a good list of choices. I enjoy drinking Yellowtail Shiraz (a rich red wine produced without animal products) while my boyfriend prefers Baba black lager, a dark vegan beer.

Snacks

Many of us like to go on dates that keep us moving. Whether we're hiking, exploring a new city, or walking around our hometown, we often find ourselves in motion and hungry for a snack.

Tracking down a plant-based snack is as easy as vegan apple pie, as long as one knows what to look for and what to watch out for. Of course there are many health food stores that sell snacks labeled vegan; big grocery stores and other shops also have a wealth of options.

Fruits, nuts, and vegetables are usually not very hard to find. One can locate them at grocery stores, out-of-the-way country stands, and even gas stations. If you're going for a hike, or will be out with your date for a long time, you may want to pack a couple of pieces of fruit and a small bag of nuts to take along. When I was hiking on the Great Wall of China, I tossed small baggies of dried fruit into my backpack each morning. Preparing in advance can save you the discomfort of being far away from home and hungry.

Packaged vegan snacks can be found in many stores, though they may not be labeled vegan. All we need to do in that case is read the ingredient list. Though it might be easy to assume a snack such as potato chips is vegan, some contain animal-derived ingredients including honey and dairy products. Our eyes are our best tools in these cases, and a quick read of the ingredients will tell us if a bag of chips passes the vegan test.

Besides the obvious non-vegan ingredients such as milk, honey, and eggs, you'll want to look for a few other animal-derived products when picking a snack. Some of the common vegan-unfriendly ingredients found in snack foods include casein (a milk protein), lactic acid (derived from milk), lactose (also made from milk), whey (another by-product of milk), carmine (a dye made from crushed insects), and gelatin (derived from animal skin and other body parts). Keep an eye out for these ingredients, as they can be found in a number of otherwise plant-based foods.

If you find yourself staring at an ingredients list and unable to decipher whether the food is vegan, you can always opt for the simplicity of an apple. But if you are determined to purchase something pre-made, there are many options.

At a major chain grocery store, I recently found a wonderful selection of vegan snacks, great for on-the-go dates. Bobo's Oat Bars, which are gluten- and soy-free, were offered in three flavors and clearly labeled vegan. Most cruelty-free items in a grocery store will not be labeled vegan, though. In another aisle, I found Ocean Spray Craisins with only two ingredients: cran-berries and sugar. Though not marked vegan, these are easy to decipher as plant-based. Large grocery stores may also sell tasty Clif "energy" bars—many of which do not contain animal products. Just read the ingredients to be sure the flavor you have picked is cruelty-free.

If you have access to a health food store or food co-op, your options may increase exponentially, as many of these establishments offer a large selection of vegan items, and the staff is likely to be knowledgeable about what is and isn't vegan. I went to a local health food store in search of vegan snacks and discovered many offerings that would be great on-the-go. Harvest Snaps are crispy, lightly salted snap peas with no animal products. I also found Emmy's dark cacao macaroons, clearly marked vegan.

Health food stores and food co-ops often have a bulk foods section, where a selection of foods—including dried fruit and nuts—can be scooped out of large bins and packaged in small baggies. The majority of these foods are usually vegan and can also be great for on-the-go snacking. Because you can scoop as much as you want, it's easy to take just a little to eat on a walk, or a lot for a weekend-long camping trip.

On the Road

I tend to favor whole foods that haven't been processed much. Brown rice, raw vegetables, chickpeas, and pumpkin seeds all make regular appearances on my plate. I feel physically and emotionally better when I eat few processed foods. However, when I go on weekend (or longer) road trips and camping adventures with my boyfriend, it can be challenging to find restaurants serving whole vegan foods on the long stretches of highway that take us to our destinations. What is a vegan gal to do for food when on a romantic out-of-the-way trip?

Traveling through unfamiliar territory with a partner, one can still find vegan meals. Large chain restaurants, frequently found near highways, have been making more and more changes to their menus that reflect a growing demand for plant-based foods. Because of their expanding options, one can count on many large chains for animal-free offerings. Chain restaurants with vegan options include Taco Bell, Chipotle, and Le Pain Quotidien. Even Dunkin' Donuts serves almond milk now, so you can secure a vegan latte at gas stations by thruways throughout the United States.

Though you may stumble upon a wonderful independent restaurant with plenty of vegan dishes while rolling down the highway, even if you don't discover that perfect place, you should still be able to find something cruelty-free to eat.

There may not be a raw vegan bistro on that long, straight stretch of road leading to your destination, but the strip mall coming up on the right might surprise you with some delicious plant-based selections.

Remember, most of these restaurants expanded their vegan options because individuals let management know that's what they wanted. If you would like to see more plant-based items at a chain restaurant, you can send them a friendly letter. You never know what might happen.

In 1992, Farm Sanctuary persuaded the Burger King near their Watkins Glen, New York, shelter to sell a veggie burger by speaking with the franchise owner Dennis Kessler. The farm animal advocacy organization then organized a grassroots call-in campaign and pushed Burger King to offer the meat-free option nationwide. The burger was so successful, and demand so great, that the massive restaurant chain began to offer it throughout the United States.

When asking a restaurant to provide plant-based options, Farm Sanctuary president and cofounder Gene Baur says, "I'd advise a gentle approach and appeal to the restaurant (owner)'s interest in selling foods that meet the demand of a growing plant-based movement. It's helpful to create mutually beneficial relationships and to support businesses that are taking positive steps in the right direction."

One person's request for foods to suit their own dietary needs can be an act of friendly activism that helps a movement.

If you are a devoted raw vegan, or would rather not eat at a chain restaurant, the ever-present grocery store has everything you need to put together a plant-based meal on the road. My mostly raw breakfasts are often composed of cherry tomatoes, baby carrots, and almonds, all of which can be found in virtually any grocery store.

There is truly nothing to fear. A committed vegan can find cruelty-free food just about anywhere one can find food. And food is just about everywhere.

Quick Guide: Vegan/Not Vegan Movie Theater Treats

Movies are a perennial date favorite. Most couples can count at least one trip to the movies in their dating histories. For many of us, our first move upon entering a theater is to head to the snack counter. But those flashy packages can be confusing when it comes to what's inside. If we were to read through all of the ingredients on each one, we might miss the start of our film. So here's a handy guide to which movie theater treats are and aren't vegan.

Movie Theater Treat	Vegan	Not Vegan
Dots	X	
Junior Mints		X
Jujyfruits	X	
M&Ms (plain, peanut)		X
Mike & Ike		X
Milk Duds		X
Skittles	X	
Swedish Fish	X	
Sour Patch Kids	X	
Twizzlers	X	

NOTE: Candy manufacturers occasionally change the recipes for their products. Check the ingredients list to be sure your favorite treat is still animal-free. Sometimes a non-vegan candy will become vegan when the producer changes its recipe. A sweet surprise!

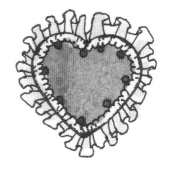

CHAPTER 8

Let's Stay Together: Cohabiting as a Vegan

Many of us who enter into long-term relationships will eventually want to move in with our partners. Though this can be a joyful and exciting moment in a romance, for those of us who are vegan, it can bring up some questions and concerns. If we are dating an omnivore, we may worry that they will bring animal products into our shared home. What if we don't want our meat-eating mate to cook their food in our pots and pans?

Sharing Your Home With Your Partner as a Vegan

As fate would have it, I landed in a living situation with a fellow vegan. It hadn't been my goal, but as it turned out, the person who I settled down with was also living a cruelty-free lifestyle.

I've found the benefits of sharing a household with a fellow vegan to be many. We don't debate about whether we purchase a down blanket (we don't), and both of us consciously try to keep animal products out of our home. Neither of us worry about opening the refrigerator door to a scene of dead animal flesh, and each of us can rest assured we won't be kissing someone who has the juice of a steak on their lips. It is comforting for me to know that our house is a cruelty-free zone.

However, not every vegan will share these values with a partner. Many of us choose to cohabit with a vegetarian or omnivore. Some of us will make a commitment to a fellow vegan, and then see that person begin to eat animal products again. Though there are a large number of vegan couples, there are also many vegan women who live with non-vegan partners.

My partner and I share various opinions and beliefs, and there are some areas where we completely disagree. This is true for many couples. Though women often look for mates who share our most strongly held values, the truth is that we will most likely disagree with our partners on some issues. What we can tolerate as far as differences is for each one of us to decide. One person might have very liberal political views and not feel comfortable in a relationship with someone who is conservative. Another person might not feel that those views are very important. In the same respect, some of us will be perfectly comfortable sharing a home with a non-vegan, and there are those of us who won't tolerate it.

When living with a partner who isn't vegan, one can try to negotiate guidelines about animal products coming into the home. Some of us won't be offended by meat in the refrigerator and non-vegan furniture in the house. However, if the presence of animal flesh and leather where you live makes you uncomfortable, you can have a conversation with your mate about it. Holding back our vegan voices to appease a partner can deny us our true selves.

I was told a story about a couple who moved in together, followed by the immediate announcement by one to the other that their new shared household would be all-vegan. How would anybody feel having a rule imposed on them in such a forceful and abrupt way? Though animal products in a home may make us feel terribly uncomfortable, there is a potentially peaceful solution. Rather than ordering our partners to play by our rules, we can sit down and talk to them ahead of moving in together to establish guidelines.

Just as we would want our partners to feel comfortable in a shared home, it's likely that our cohabitants will want us to be at ease, too. When we speak from the "I" perspective, we do not accuse or label our loved one. So we can say, "I feel uncomfortable when I open up the refrigerator and see meat" or, "I would feel so much better in a home without leather or down, can we talk about alternatives?"

If we let go of trying to control our partner's responses, and accept whatever they might say, we won't be disappointed if they don't agree with our requests.

Many people who are vegan would prefer not to have meat in the house, but simply accept it as a reality. If we feel violated in a home that contains dead animal flesh, and are unable to negotiate a comfortable situation, perhaps we shouldn't move into that household.

If one becomes vegan while already living with an omnivore, there's still the possibility of establishing guidelines. You can have that same conversation with a partner you are currently cohabiting with. Accusing a partner of doing things we deem "bad," or launching into a speech about cruelty to animals probably won't help, but explaining, "I would feel much better if we kept our pots separate," might lead to an agreeable arrangement.

You may not be able to keep a perfectly vegan household when living with an omnivore, but are any vegans truly perfect? Even if your request for a meat-free fridge is denied, you may be able to find some middle ground. Perhaps you could purchase a second refrigerator to keep your food in. Or use separate dishes and silverware, so that you can be confident they haven't touched meat.

In the end, though we love and respect our partners and want them to be happy, there's no reason to do that at the expense of our own feelings of comfort. If we've had the conversations and can find no compromise, it may be time to look inside ourselves and decide how much we can tolerate. If it is so painful to be in our home, do we really want to stay there?

But before you move out, just remember that time after time, meat-eaters have shifted toward a plant-based diet as the result of loving and living with a cruelty-free gal. Being our healthy, happy, compassionate selves is one of the best forms of advocacy and service to the animals. I have spoken with many women who accepted an omnivore partner, only to be happily surprised when that person began to eat fewer animal products. If you live with an omnivore and cook amazing plant-based meals, they may become more and more open to your lifestyle. By simply living compassionately, gently sharing your knowledge, and having an abundance of delicious animal-free food in the house, you may influence a cohabitant toward the vegan end of the spectrum.

When we fall in love with someone, we often turn a blind eye to their values that are different than our own. This can be easy to do when we're not spending most of our time with them. Eventually, however, we may want to share a home with that person, or cohabit.

Living with someone you love can be a wonderful experience, but it can also come with some new stresses. How to split the bills, who will do the dishes, and which one of you is going to take out the garbage are all topics likely to come up. For vegans, one of these concerns may be rules about animal products in the home.

Some vegan women are happiest cohabiting with a fellow vegan, and that's what they stick with, but many live with an omnivore.

In mixed (one vegan and one non-vegan) partnerships, the women (and men) I spoke with said their relationships worked best when the vegan extended their circle of compassion to the person they lived with—not forcing rules, nor pressuring their partner to change. In more cases than not, those omnivore cohabitants began to cut out the cruelty, eating fewer animal products.

The vegan women I spoke with who committed to living with omnivores extended their love to those people while staying strong in their own compassionate lifestyles. And in most cases, other humans began to live more compassionately because of the vegans in their lives.

Everybody Has Their Moment
JL Fields, Writer, Consultant, Vegan Cook,
Lifestyle Coach, and Educator

The author of *Vegan Pressure Cooking,* and coauthor of *Vegan for Her*, JL Fields has supported many on their compassionate paths as a coach, educator, author, host of the *Easy Vegan* radio show, and board member for more than one animal rights nonprofit organization.

I spoke to JL early on in the writing of this book about her experiences being married to an omnivorous husband.

JL had shifted to a vegan diet in 2010, initially for health reasons. However, once she stopped eating animal products, she started to learn more about the egregious conditions animals farmed for food are subject to, and other ways they suffer. "I went vegan and then started to learn things," she says, "and . . . visited a farm animal sanctuary. I'm like, I totally get it." Though she had initially switched to a plant-based diet to benefit her body, she became an ethical vegan, motivated by her desire to curb cruelty to animals.

For JL, sharing a home with a husband who ate animals was not a problem, as they had both always maintained their individuality in the relationship. When JL became a Buddhist, her husband, Dave, respected her choice, and she didn't pressure him to make the same change. Two years later, he became a Buddhist on his own. She took the same approach when she became vegan.

Living with an omnivore husband did not prevent JL from expressing her interest and excitement about veganism to him, and she frequently shared her passion about that part of her life. He supported her in her enthusiasm, although he didn't choose that path for himself. JL was comfortable in a home that wasn't completely vegan. "Do we use the same pots and pans? Absolutely," she said.

There were some major shifts along the way, however. "We were at an event in Manhattan a few months ago," said JL, "and they showed a brief documentary . . . on how down is produced, and you literally saw someone pull the feathers out of the chest of a goose." Dave immediately decided he would no longer purchase any products containing down. "Every single step he does, that's all a victory," she shared. "I am totally supportive of that."

JL's philosophy about people becoming vegan is that everybody has their moment. Most human beings have a love of animals in their hearts. And many vegans have had a moment that inspired their commitment to a cruelty-free lifestyle. "I had a moment," said JL. "He will have his moment."

And he did.

I spoke to JL again, two years after our initial conversation, and she had some news to share.

When the couple moved from New York City to Colorado Springs, Colorado, JL's husband surprised her with a suggestion that they make their new home vegetarian. "So at that point there was no more meat in the house," says JL, "and when we bought new things . . . we didn't have down . . ." A few months later, the pair moved into a new home, and Dave suggested they make it all vegan.

"He just made that decision on his own," says JL. "He shocked me."

The following year, JL invited Dave to try a three-week program of vegan eating, which she would guide him in. He agreed, and during the last weekend of the experiment, they went to see the film *Cowspiracy*, about the massive negative impact of animal farming on the environment. "When we were driving home from Denver to Colorado Springs that night, he looked at me and he said, 'I know you're vegan for the animals, I've never connected to it in that way, but tonight I got it,'" says JL. "He went vegan."

"Well, I've got to tell you, in the car it just blew me away," she says about Dave's sudden shift.

Not only is Dave now vegan, but he makes it clear to others that they have a cruelty-free household and that animal products are not permitted. "It just brings me immense joy that my partner takes pride in our vegan home," says JL.

When I first spoke to her two years ago, JL offered that though vegan women might prefer dating only those who shared their lifestyle, it might be hard to find a partner within that limited pool. "I don't look at people as non-vegans," she had said. "I look at people as they are not vegan yet, and I'm just going to live my happy, joyful vegan life and hope that it has some kind of impact. And I would probably give that advice to people who are dating. Don't judge someone for where they are but also don't assume they're going to change because then you're all going to be set up for disappointment. Just know that we're all on a journey and what is right now might not be the way it is a year from now."

If you can accept that your partner is an omnivore and love that person for who they are—acknowledging that they, too, may (or may not) have their moment—you could find peace living with someone who is different than you. And that omnivore might someday become a vegan.

Different Diets Don't Break Their Bond
Jen Albanese, Medical Biller at a Hospital

Deeply devoted to the animals, Jen Albanese is proudly vegan and also spends hours each week volunteering at a no-kill cat and dog shelter near her Cold Spring, New York, home. Though her husband does not share her vegan lifestyle, Jen is unwavering in her commitment to help animals by eschewing animal products.

She went vegan in 1994. "I just couldn't take it anymore," Jen says. She was disgusted by the meat and dairy industries and says the cruelties of farming were causing her to be depressed. She wanted to take actions in her life to stop the suffering. "I just did it without thinking twice, and it was so easy, and I felt so good . . . I felt clean and happy," she says about going vegan.

Jen was already married to her omnivore husband at the time she went vegan, so they needed to negotiate a household that previously had no rules concerning animal products. "In the beginning," she says, "I would still prepare his food, but it wouldn't bother me . . . because I wasn't eating the animals." After some time had passed, Jen told her husband that she could no longer tolerate cooking meat. Following their conversation, "I would prepare food that was vegan," says Jen, "and if he wanted a piece of meat, he'd have to cook it himself outside on the grill." Her husband amicably agreed to the arrangement.

Her husband has never disparaged Jen in any way for her vegan lifestyle. "That's one thing, I really doubt we'd be together today if he ever disrespected me, or made fun of me about that. I wouldn't go for that."

With the exception of food, Jen's husband agrees to keep their household as vegan as possible. "There's nothing in our house that is animal skin, or fur, or down," she says.

Though she would prefer that her husband eat an entirely plant-based diet, Jen has seen him move in that direction, consuming more vegan food and fewer animal products. "He's very open-minded . . . he'll try everything," she says, "which . . . satisfies me for now." Jen adds that the amount of meat and dairy in their household has decreased over the years since she went vegan. She speaks to her husband on a regular basis about the cruelties of animal farming, keeping in mind that he might one day opt to become vegan himself, but staying aware that he may not.

Jen and her husband don't see eye to eye on veganism, however they have a strong relationship that holds them together despite their differences. She appreciates the changes he has made and stays strong in her own commitments to the animals, even if he doesn't share them. Her husband respects her needs as a vegan and has never challenged or insulted her lifestyle. Together they peacefully coexist, one a devoted vegan, the other an omnivore.

Jen believes vegans and omnivores can live together in harmony, "but always educate them about the animals used for food and products," she says. "Hopefully it will have an impact on them to change, even if it's a small change."

Books Brought Them Together, and to Veganism
Colleen Patrick-Goudreau, Author, Speaker, and Host
of the Food for Thought podcast
David Goudreau, Software Consultant

The celebrated author of seven books about vegan cooking and cruelty-free living, as well as host of the incredibly popular *Food for Thought* podcast, Colleen Patrick-Goudreau has inspired many people to choose a compassionate lifestyle and has helped them along their paths. She provides crucial information, advice, insights, and recipes in a matter-of-fact, yet gentle manner. Colleen communicates the benefits of veganism in a very personal way and speaks to podcast listeners in the voice of a sensible friend. She reminds us that in our hearts most of us don't want to hurt others, and to follow that inner compass. I personally became hooked on Colleen's podcasts long before I went vegan, and listening helped see me through the transition. In other words, I am a fan.

Colleen, who lives in Oakland, California, with her husband, David, originally went vegan in 1998, when the two were cohabiting but not yet married. She had stopped eating land animals eight years prior in response to reading John Robbins's revelatory book *Diet for a New America*. At age twenty-eight, she again read a book that changed her outlook, *Slaughterhouse*, and immediately converted to a vegan lifestyle. The book explained in no uncertain terms that farming animals for their eggs and milk is a cruel and exploitative industry. Reading it, Colleen learned of the violence inherent in farming animals for these secretions and realized that she was contributing to it by consuming them. It's not surprising that Colleen, who has a master's degree in English literature and met her partner working in a bookstore, came to live a cruelty-free lifestyle in response to reading books. As opposed to "becoming a vegan," Colleen saw the process more as becoming true to herself. She says, "[A]ll the blocks to all the compassion that was already inside me were just dismantled, and that's what becoming vegan meant for me . . ."

Colleen was away from home when she read *Slaughterhouse*, and having such a strong response, called David. "I just said, 'I'm vegan, and I can't have any of this in my house, it's just too upsetting. I can't even look at it.'" David completely accepted and supported Colleen's commitment. "He was like, 'Okay sweetheart, your happiness is more important than me having shrimp in the freezer.'" David agreed to an animal product–free home, so there was no conflict when it came to household items. About six months later, David was inspired by Colleen to read the same books she had read and he embraced veganism for himself, too.

Says David, "When Colleen first told me that she was going vegan it was not an issue for me at all. In fact, I was very open to the possibilities because I saw it as a personal choice of hers and felt that if this was important to her, the best thing I could do was to be open to it and supportive of it . . . I didn't feel threatened at all."

Colleen didn't pressure David to read any of the books she had read, nor to be vegan. His joining Colleen in her lifestyle grew organically out of their relationship—about which Colleen says, "we inspire one another." She adds, "If I read a book, any book that's meaningful, or see a movie that's meaningful, I want to share it with people, and especially the people I love . . . I think it was really important for him to read the books himself, and he did, and that's when he became vegan."

Colleen shares that when David went vegan, "It deepened our relationship and certainly deepened my affection for him." She has said on her podcast, "What attracted me to David was that he was open, loving, kind, intelligent, compassionate, and thoughtful—and those are all pretty much the prerequisites for and the foundation of being vegan." She says, "I think we come together to inspire each other to be better in this world . . . David didn't become vegan for me nor did I 'convert him.' I was inspired and moved and changed by some things I had read, and I asked him if he would read them, too . . . I brought him the information, but it was the information itself that moved him."

A Life-Changing Campout
Robyn Moore, Humane Educator
Martin Moore, Program Director for a Research and Development Group

Forty-one-year-old New Yorker Robyn Moore is an outspoken activist who educates others about veganism through her *Raising Veg Kids* website, and by organizing the children's area at the New York City Vegetarian Food Festival. Her calm and mild manner invites listeners, young and old, to pay attention, learn, and ask questions.

However, when she arrived at veganism in 2006 after attending an animal rights conference that educated her about the cruelties of farming animals, her omnivore husband, Martin, was not eager to hear about it. "I didn't get it and I argued with her about it," he explains.

Though Robyn had been a vegetarian since the age of thirteen, the switch to veganism represented a major shift in her awareness and thinking. Prior to the conference, she says, "I didn't have any idea about what went on in the dairy industry, or egg industry." She left the event "feeling really sad and traumatized, but also inspired to make a difference." Within three weeks she was vegan.

Robyn's husband, Martin, questioned what Robyn had been told that had upset her so much: "I just wasn't supportive of the vegan concept, and I didn't understand what it was all about. And actually, even more than that, I disagreed with the concept." He wasn't aware at the time of the mistreatment suffered by the vast majority of animals who are farmed for food.

Martin recalls being challenged by Robyn's switch to veganism. "I think when she was a vegetarian, I don't think it really was that big a deal. . . . It was actually pretty easy from what I remember." But Martin found cohabiting with a vegan difficult. "When she went vegan, then it was definitely more of a bigger contrast to what I was eating . . . it was more of an effort for her and for me." He adds, "I didn't get it and I argued with her about it." Martin didn't like that the vegan philosophy was so prominent at every meal.

Martin was convinced that the fault lay with those who were sharing information with Robyn and was frustrated with them for upsetting her. "It sounded like a wild scare tactic," he says.

Robyn explains, "It was hard for me to understand how such a compassionate, reasonable, smart person with so much integrity could not understand the ramifications of what he was eating, or even want to know where it came from."

Then Robyn extended an invitation. The pair had recently purchased camping gear for a trip to Iceland under the condition that they use the equipment again. So Robyn asked her husband to go camping at Farm Sanctuary's shelter in Watkins Glen, New York. She suggested the two attend the organization's annual Hoe Down, a weekend of talks by experts and visits with the rescued animals who live there. Martin agreed to the trip, thinking that he would skip the talks.

He ate a hamburger at McDonald's on the way to the event—it would be his last.

Once at Farm Sanctuary, Martin was struck by the diverse group of people he met who were opposed to factory farming. He was also impressed by the delicious vegan food. He decided that since the other attendees seemed reasonable, he would sit in on some of the talks, which were being given by animal rights leaders including philosopher and author Peter Singer. Martin listened to the simple facts of factory farms, saw the cages that pigs are confined in, and learned about the tiny amount of space chickens are given to live out their lives.

Martin also spent time with some of the rescued animals who live at the sanctuary. He saw how distorted their bodies are from the factory farming industry's manipulations. He had met many animals who lived on farms when he was growing up, but had not previously seen those whose bodies had been bred to be so misshapen that "almost their very existence is painful and difficult," he says. The bodies of the animals he met now had been altered in this way only for the sake of producing more food.

Martin left the Hoe Down thinking, *if what I was being told about animal treatment was really true, and as widespread as these people are saying, then I won't be able to support it.* He says, "I actually effectively went vegan immediately."

Robyn's husband followed the informative weekend with his own research into the issues, further cementing his commitment to veganism. He explains that nothing Robyn could have said to him would have convinced him to stop eating animal products, and that he had to find his own path to a cruelty-free lifestyle.

"I didn't bring him to the Hoe Down thinking that I was going to change him," says Robyn. When they left Farm Sanctuary, "We really didn't talk about it very much. I didn't want to push it," she explains. However, Martin's views had shifted, and not too much later he shared with Robyn that he was now vegan.

"When I was vegan, and Martin wasn't," says Robyn, "I felt hurt, angry, and confused. When I learned about how much animals suffer on factory farms, of course I wanted to share it with him." But speaking to her husband about the issues did not encourage him. "So when I began this journey, and he wasn't ready to embark on the same journey, it felt like we were missing something. The relationship was at a standstill for those few months," she says. "Veganism was one of the most important decisions in my life, and it felt like he just didn't get it. That was hard. Luckily, it only took about four months for him to 'get it,' and our relationship was back on track. Now we're on the same journey, one that follows the path of compassion and integrity. And we have two sweet kids along for the ride!"

Setting a Powerful Example
Cynthia King, Artistic Director of Cynthia King Dance Studio and Founder of Cynthia King Vegan Ballet Slippers

Cynthia King is a strong voice for the animals and a devoted vegan who has carried her activism into her work. She created the world's first line of ready-to-wear vegan ballet slippers, which are now required footwear at her studio and worn by dancers around the globe. She has also choreographed elaborate dance pieces to shed light on issues including factory farming and the cruelty of circuses.

Cynthia first met her husband, Rodney—an omnivore at the time—in 1986, and the two married in 1990. She had become aware of animal suffering at an early age, committing to vegetarianism at ten years old, and later going vegan.

Because of their dietary differences, when they married and moved in together, the two each cooked for themselves. With very different schedules, often working opposite shifts, it was easy for them to each be responsible for their own meals. The couple did, however, agree that no meat be cooked in the pots and pans that Cynthia used.

For the most part, Cynthia was able to address any discomfort around living in a non-vegan household in this way, though she explains that, "If I smelled meat cooking, I would be disgusted." She says she quietly wished that her husband might go vegetarian, but never pressured him to do so.

Six years into their marriage, something changed. Months after the couple's first son, Major, was born, Rodney revealed to Cynthia that he was now vegetarian. "I didn't even notice it," says Cynthia, "because we mostly had meals separately." Rodney told Cynthia that he had made the switch because he knew their son wouldn't be eating meat and wanted them to be more of a family.

Though Cynthia never tried to convince Rodney to eat differently, she says, "When he stopped eating meat, I was happy and relieved."

Later, her husband took even greater steps to lessen the suffering in his diet and today Cynthia, Rodney, and their two teenage sons, Major and Jet, are all vegan.

Rodney not only stopped eating animal products, but became a strong advocate for plant-based eating at his place of work. "I know a lot of people who became vegetarian and vegan under his guidance. He was very vocal about it at his job," Cynthia says.

Cynthia proudly shares that Major has also been spreading the vegan love. "My son's girlfriend became vegan (and an activist) about a year after they began dating. Be still my heart!"

"I think that often the most effective form of activism is simply being a powerful example to those around you," says Cynthia. "This goes for dating, socializing, anytime you're interacting with others. When people notice your principles in action, and see how easy it is to live and let live, this goes a long way."

By living boldly, strongly, and compassionately, while remaining tolerant of those different than herself, Cynthia has inspired her family, and many others, to cut the cruelty out of their lives.

Moving in the Same Direction
Liz Levine, Sales and Marketing Professional
Mitchell Rigie, Founder and Partner of a Training
and Development Company

When New Yorker Liz Levine went vegan, she had no expectation that her omnivore husband, Mitchell, would follow suit. Says Mitchell, "I gotta tell you, she was very clear and just said, 'Look, you don't have to change anything, this is just for me . . .'" Liz let Mitchell know that her commitment to veganism was about shifts in her own lifestyle, and she had no intention of convincing him to adjust the way he ate, too. But he did.

Like many, Liz arrived at veganism both because of her love of animals, and her desire to eat more healthily. She was aware of the cruelties of factory farming and had also come to believe that her diet, highly reliant on animal proteins, was to her detriment. When she decided to try veganism, she thought, *I want to see how I feel because I don't think this high [animal] protein thing is working for me at all.*

Liz started to cut the cruelty out of her lifestyle by switching to a vegan diet, and later began to phase out animal products in other areas of her life, such as her clothes. At first she was challenged by trying to think of dinner as a proper meal without meat, but she soon discovered the benefits of eating plant-based. "I realized that I actually had a lot more stamina," she says.

Initially nervous about how her husband might react to her ethical overhaul, Liz discovered that he was completely supportive. Her concerns that her dietary shift would drive them apart proved unfounded. Mitchell explains that Liz's evolution into eating more humanely was a natural progression, given her deep empathy for animals. "He had a good foundation for who I was," Liz says.

Not only was Liz's new lifestyle not divisive, but husband Mitchell became inspired to move in her direction. After the couple visited Farm Sanctuary, and watched a few documentaries that addressed the cruelties of animal agriculture, he committed to eating a much more plant-based diet, bringing the couple closer together, rather than driving them apart.

Liz didn't pressure Mitchell to follow her lead, nor did she consciously try to convince him. However, she found that both he and his daughter were quick to jump on board. For the first few weeks of her new lifestyle, Liz purchased meat for her family, but soon her stepdaughter voiced concern, pleading with Liz not to buy it again. "[She] said something so profound," Liz shares, repeating her stepdaughter's words, "I want to eat what you're eating. I don't want to kill an animal if I don't have to."

Prior to Mitchell's change in diet, he, like Liz, had been eating a great deal of animal products. "I was having three eggs every morning, chicken for lunch, and some big animal protein for dinner almost exclusively," he explains. "The only things I kept were the eggs in the morning. Occasionally I'll have fish, but not so often."

"It wasn't as hard as I thought it was going to be," says Mitchell. "I can't see going back."

Liz attributes Mitchell's change to doing what was best for herself. It is "attraction, not promotion," she says, that has worked in her relationship. By simply living her own truth, those who she loved followed suit. She says, "Leading by example has never failed me . . . You know that's very contagious. It's very powerful." She adds, "I think allowing the people in your house to make their own choices is such a respectful way to go about it."

Liz encourages vegans living with omnivore partners to understand that their mates may not share their values. "I think it's very important to remember that you're having this awakening, but maybe your partner is not having that going on for them right now," she says. Liz and Mitchell have shown that by simply following what one knows is best for them, even the most devoted omnivore partner may become inspired to make a compassionate shift.

A Growing Circle of Compassion
Autumn Williams-Wussow, Early Childhood Teacher

Thirty-six-year-old Autumn Williams-Wussow lives in Beacon, New York, with her wife, Jennie, and their young son, Bay. She came to veganism as a teenager after growing up in a vegetarian household. At first a hamburger-eating child, when she was about seven years old Autumn's mother announced that their home would now be completely meat-free. So it wasn't a giant leap when she went vegan as a teenager and started the animal rights club at her high school. Her family followed her lead, and soon the entire household was eating cruelty-free.

Autumn has been in two major relationships in her life; one while in college, and now with her wife (who she has been involved with for the past ten years). In each case, Autumn's partner entered the relationship a meat-eater and came to eat a more plant-based diet.

Autumn and her wife met as activists working for the common cause of addressing sexual violence. However, when it came to animal rights, they were of two minds.

Autumn says that before she made a commitment to omnivore Jennie, she had thought she'd prefer to be in a relationship with a vegan. "I could see the value of being with somebody who had the same thoughts about eating animals," but, she says, "I fell in love."

"We would go out to eat all the time," says Autumn, "and she was ordering meat back in the day, when we first got together, quite a bit. And I think it did bother me."

Though Autumn had grown up in a supportive vegetarian, and then vegan, household, Jennie's homelife had been much different. "She was raised super meat and potatoes," says Autumn.

Autumn dealt with her discomfort around her partner's meat-eating by talking to her about it. "We had conversations."

Jennie slowly came to eat a more plant-based diet. When the two moved in together two years into their relationship, they chose not to keep meat in their home. A few years later, Jennie told Autumn that the only meat she would continue to eat was fish. "These were things that she [did] slowly, and it wasn't necessarily something she was talking about all the time," but through the years, Autumn's wife took clear steps to curb the cruelty in her diet.

Autumn explains that living an example of a happy, healthy, cruelty-free life is probably what inspired Jennie's changes the most.

However, Jennie made the decision to eat more humanely for herself, not in an effort to appease Autumn. "I check in with her," says Autumn. "I'm like, 'Are you doing this because I want you to, or are you doing this because you want to?' and she says, 'Because I want to,' so that's nice."

Though Jennie still eats some animal products, the couple easily agreed to raise their son vegan.

Autumn is happy about Jennie's shift toward a more plant-based diet, but she still experiences difficult feelings when Jennie eats animal products, like when she orders a latte with cow's milk. "It really does affect me. It makes me sad," says Autumn.

When faced with those uncomfortable moments, Autumn tries to tap into the same love that she feels for the animals. She aims to extend her circle of compassion to her wife, even when her partner is making choices Autumn doesn't agree with. "Everyone's in their own place, everyone's where they are now, and you can't push anybody," says Autumn.

In addition to eating a more plant-based diet, Jennie has minimized her use of animal products in other areas of her life. Though she continues to use non-vegan items she already owns, such as a down comforter, "There's an assumption that she wouldn't buy new products," says Autumn. "She has stopped buying leather shoes, but it wasn't because of any house rules we talked about. I think it's part of her gradual exploration of possibilities beyond animal products as she is exposed to [the] vegan lifestyle."

As Autumn continues to follow her own strong vegan path, she has found that slowly but surely, Jennie has been taking her own steps in a cruelty-free direction.

Tips For Coexistence: Suggestions For Peaceful Cohabitation

Many omnivores admire their vegan partners for their ethical lifestyles. However, creating a vegan-friendly household may take some negotiating.

Some vegans will be comfortable with a cohabitant bringing animal products into the household, and some will not. All we can do is listen to our hearts and gauge our limitations by how we feel.

If you feel too uncomfortable to cook your dinner in a pan used for meat, or you can't bear to have down blankets in your household, you can have a conversation with your loved one. Chances are they want you to be happy in your own home.

When we speak from the "I" perspective, we avoid denying our partners their own feelings. By letting go of expectations, we lower our risk of disappointment. In being gentle, and not accusatory, we avoid prompting a defensive response.

Here are some examples of situations you might run into, and what you might say to address them:

Issue: The soap your partner just bought for the bathroom was made with goat's milk, and it's making you sick to your stomach.
You say: I really appreciate that you picked up bathroom supplies, but I feel uncomfortable with soap made out of goat's milk. Can we choose something together that we both like?

Issue: You've been vegan for some time now and are no longer comfortable with your partner cooking steak in the same pan that you use for tofu.
You say: I want to be sure to prepare my food in pots and pans that haven't touched animal products. Why don't I buy my own set that we can keep separate from the rest?

Issue: You want to share cooking duties with your partner, but they have requested meat at every meal.

You say: For me, cooking meat would go against my ethics, and it would be painful for me to cook it, but I'm happy to prepare delicious vegan food for you.

Issue: You and your partner have decided to purchase a new couch but your cohabitant is eyeing one that has down in it.

You say: I'm excited that we're buying a new sofa together but won't feel comfortable sitting on one that has down. There are so many cruelty-free alternatives. I'd love to go shopping with you for something that's made without animal products.

Issue: Your partner's mother just walked into the housewarming party in your cruelty-free home and handed you a tray of fruit and (non-vegan) cheese.

You say (as kindly and gently as possible): Thank you so much for coming to our party, and thinking to bring something. We're so happy you're here. We love fruit and cheese but we're keeping a vegan home, so I'll put this wonderful fruit out with some great vegan cheese.

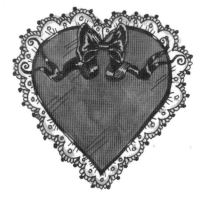

CHAPTER 9

It's a Nice Day For a Veg Wedding: A Compassionate Celebration

Like many other little girls, when I was growing up, I imagined a grand wedding, with a big white gown, a groom in a tuxedo, and a long aisle framed by guests craning their necks to see me. I don't know when, but somehow, at some point, that dream dissipated, and I learned that there are no rules when it comes to weddings. A wedding can be anything we want it to be.

Today, though I still dream of wedding dresses, I imagine a nuptial celebration that isn't necessarily all about me and what I'm wearing, but about love. Love for my partner, love for my friends and family, and love and compassion for animals. As a vegan, I would want a completely cruelty-free wedding, perhaps set at a farm animal sanctuary.

Many elements of a wedding have traditionally not been vegan. What about those meaty main courses? Egg-heavy wedding cakes? And makeup artists wielding carmine-containing lipsticks?

Just as with restaurants, clothing, and cosmetics, creating a vegan wedding means making compassionate choices. One may not be able to work with any caterer in the world, select from every dress in the bridal shop, or choose just any cake baker, but wouldn't we be selective about these elements anyway? Most brides wouldn't consider wearing just any dress or serving whatever cake happened to be available. The difference in having a vegan wedding is that our criteria includes kindness to animals.

When we close the door on cruelty in planning a wedding, we discover yet again that taking the compassionate route provides us with wonderful options. It may take a little extra work, but the reward of having a vegan wedding is knowing that our union with our loved one didn't cost anyone their lives. A wedding, after all, is a celebration of love, so in planning that day, wouldn't we want to honor our love for all beings?

Venues

As vegans, we have a wide selection of wedding venues to pick from. There are many lovely locations that fit the cruelty-free bill. These include animal sanctuaries, community gardens, Victorian mansions, and mountain houses. If a venue requires that you use their caterer, you may want to check that they cannot only accommodate a vegan menu, but serve fantastic plant-based food. Some people have discovered at tastings that a caterer offering vegan dishes may only provide rudimentary options, leaving engaged couples feeling as flat as the steamed zucchini on their plates. If you are married to the idea of working with a particular venue that has an in-house caterer, you can offer to provide them with recipes from a favorite vegan cookbook.

Some couples opt to incorporate their love of animals into their wedding by holding it at a farm animal sanctuary. At these peaceful shelters, we are surrounded by the animals we are helping by being vegan. Also, the money one spends on a farm sanctuary venue directly benefits the animals who live at the shelter. There are farm animal sanctuaries throughout the United States and around the world, many of which will accommodate vegan weddings. Farm Sanctuary's spacious and serene animal shelter in Watkins Glen, New York, makes for a dreamy wedding locale in the heart of the Finger Lakes region. Piebird Farm Sanctuary in Nipissing, Ontario, offers vegan catering in addition to a lovely setting where guests can meet rescued animals. Opting for a farm sanctuary is a wonderful way to introduce guests to veganism by letting them spend time with the animals. Looking for something local?

Reach out to your nearest sanctuary. Even if they haven't previously hosted a wedding, you may find them receptive to your request.

For those looking to avoid a required in-house caterer, there are a number of options. When Olivia and Marie Nguyen got married, they opted for an orchard and brought in their favorite vegan caterer. This provided them with a beautiful outdoor location that celebrated nature and didn't involve any animal cruelty.

Gardens are everywhere. Even in gigantic, bustling cities like New York, community and botanical gardens can have a strong presence. Saying your vows surrounded by beautiful and fragrant flowers could be the perfect setting for your nuptials. Growing up in Manhattan, I fantasized about holding my wedding ceremony at New York City's incredible Conservatory Garden in Central Park, which only charges a $400 fee. You may be able to secure permission to wed in a community garden for free. Of course, a wedding and reception in a large botanical garden would be a pricier option. Whether in your backyard, or in the middle of a metropolis, gardens can be a beautiful setting for your big day.

Caterers

Delicious, creatively prepared plant-based food is an appetizing element of any wedding, but can also be a great way to introduce omnivore guests to veganism. A vegan wedding will often be a guest's first introduction to fine vegan dining, so it's an opportunity to show them how great it can be.

Finding a caterer for a vegan wedding may seem like a difficult task, but there are plenty of options. Even the brides I interviewed who held their weddings in sparsely populated areas were able to serve delicious plant-based food.

There are many vegan caterers these days, including revered restaurants such as Candle Cafe, and famous chefs including Jay Astafa. If you don't live in an area that boasts numerous vegan caterers, fear not, you can still have a wonderful cruelty-free wedding.

If there is no all-vegan caterer available to you, you may want to enlist a restaurant that already has vegan options on its menu. If you have a favorite

Indian restaurant that prepares its food without ghee (dairy-derived) then they may be an ideal choice. Many Thai dishes are also easily made vegan—perhaps you can work with your favorite local spot to prepare an all-vegan menu. Do you have a favorite place for dinner? They may be able to cater your wedding.

Sometimes we find the perfect wedding venue only to discover they have an in-house caterer that must be enlisted for the event. The required caterer may offer vegan options, but might not have the culinary know-how to prepare the truly special plant-based dishes you envision for your wedding. Some couples have dealt with this situation by offering the caterer a favorite vegan cookbook. Working with a non-vegan caterer can be a learning process for both parties, but just because it may require some work doesn't mean it's time to abandon all hope. Communicating with your caterer about your ideas and needs can be valuable to all involved, and many chefs are excited by the challenge of learning to prepare plant-based dishes.

When a wedding venue has a required caterer, there will generally be a tasting prior to the confirmation of your booking. If you attend the tasting and discover that their best attempt at a plant-based meal is only mediocre, you may be able to work with them to develop a more impressive menu. If not, it's fine to move on. There are many possible places to hold your wedding and other options for food.

Wedding Cakes

The baking and decorating of wedding cakes is truly an edible art form. Wedding cakes are created in every size, shape, flavor, and color imaginable. Though not all of us will require a wedding cake as part of our special day, many of us will want to make it a focal point.

There was a time when cruelty-free wedding cakes were difficult to come by. When vegan bride Kirsti Gholson (who we'll also meet later in this chapter) got married in 2002, finding a baker to create a vegan cake was so challenging, she decided to make it herself, with help from the couple's family. But today, acquiring a vegan wedding cake is not so difficult. There are plenty of bakers who will create a plant-based cake, including a growing number of all-vegan establishments. Erin McKenna's Bakery is 100 percent vegan and can provide wedding cakes that are also gluten-free out of their three locations in New York City, Los Angeles, and Orlando, Florida. The good news is that even if you are not local to one of these storefronts, the cakes can be shipped anywhere in the United States as separate pieces and assembled by your wedding's caterer. If you can't find a local vegan bakery, don't have the resources to assemble a cake, and are craving the polish of a professional, try calling shops near your venue. Many non-vegan bakeries will be able to provide you with the cruelty-free cake of your dreams if you just ask.

Wedding Attire

On her wedding day, a bride can truly wear anything. The classic gown is always an option, but not a necessity. Many women feel much more comfortable in a suit. Some ladies will opt for something colorful as opposed to traditional white. The sky is the limit when it comes to what to wear for a wedding. Just like on a date, we want to be sure our outfits on the big day reflect who we really are.

Dresses

When we think of traditional wedding dresses we tend to imagine silk (not vegan) gowns. And the truth is that most high-priced wedding dresses are, in fact, built of silk. But there are many cruelty-free options, among them gowns made of cotton, synthetic taffeta, linen, or non-silk chiffon.

Of course, as vegans, we want to stay away from any dresses that incorporate leather, fur, pearls, or feathers. These are generally a little easier to avoid than silk. Steering clear of fabrics that are animal-derived, we have the privilege of walking down the aisle knowing that animals didn't suffer for our dresses. And who wants suffering to be a part of their wedding? Even with silk out of the picture, there are still many beautiful wedding gowns to choose from.

Two names are nearly synonymous with wedding dresses, Kleinfeld and Vera Wang. The basis of a popular reality TV series—*Say Yes to the Dress*—

Kleinfeld Bridal in New York City has a long tradition of dressing brides, offering them the individual attention they crave. Many daydream of shopping for a wedding dress at this storied store.

Like Kleinfeld, a dress by designer Vera Wang is the focus of many bridal fantasies. I have to admit, I've dreamt of wearing a Vera Wang wedding gown.

I emailed Kleinfeld to see what options they might offer for vegans, inquiring if they sold any dresses that were made of completely synthetic or other vegan-appropriate fabrics. The response was, "No, sorry!" So, if you're planning a vegan wedding, Kleinfeld may not be in the cards. That's okay; you can find that personal attention elsewhere.

When I called one of Vera Wang's boutiques, I was informed that they didn't carry any silk-free wedding gowns, and custom-made dresses started at $100,000. But being vegan doesn't mean you can't buy one of the designer's gowns. If only a Vera Wang dress will do, there are not only vegan options, but they are priced lower than the designer's standard silk gowns. The David's Bridal website and stores offer a selection of nicely priced Vera Wang wedding dresses that are made out of synthetic materials, and therefore suitable for vegans. In fact, the chain of discount stores offers many gowns that can be confirmed vegan by checking their tags or descriptions at the website. David's Bridal also offers their ethical standards for review at their website, for those who want to ensure the dresses meet their requirements.

Many small bridal boutiques also offer gowns made out of synthetic materials in a range of prices. However, it's not necessary to go the traditional bridal route when picking a dress. When we let go of our old ideas about wedding dresses, the door opens to the wonderful independent designers who offer vegan-friendly bridal gowns. Or, alternately, dresses that were not intended for brides at all.

The Cotton Bride creates simple, elegant, graceful wedding gowns that, true to the company's name, are primarily made of cotton. "There is a widespread fallacy that certain fabrics are not appropriate for bridal gown design," says Fikre S. Ayele, owner and president of The Cotton Bride. Fikre explains, "Not only is cotton the primary fabric we use, but as we custom-make most of our gowns, we allow our brides to choose whatever fabric they are most comfortable with."

Tara Lynn Bridal also makes gorgeous vegan-friendly wedding dresses. The designer's Maya and Aphrodite gowns are both made of hemp and cotton, and any dress in the designer's collection may be created vegan to order. Many of Tara Lynn's dresses also incorporate color, including beautiful bright hand embroidery. The designer creates each pattern and gown by hand in her Sutton, Vermont, studio, so one can walk down the aisle confident that her dress was ethically made. Her pieces are nicely priced, with the Mariana dress costing only $600.

Don't forget: you don't have to limit yourself to dresses deemed "bridal." One of my close friends found her perfect gown in the women's section of a department store. Just be sure to check those tags to confirm the outfit in question doesn't contain animal products.

Suits and Tuxedos

Some women will opt out of a gown and in for a suit. However, most suits contain wool—not vegan! For cruelty-free brides seeking out a wedding-appropriate suit, there are also a number of options.

Brave GentleMan offers high-quality vegan clothes, traditionally worn by men, such as handsome vegan suits, that are perfect for a wedding.

In addition to gowns, Tara Lynn Bridal also designs vegan suits, including a hemp option that is perfect for the bride who wouldn't ever consider wearing a dress. Brides looking to complete their look may opt for one of the designer's sweet bow ties.

Vegan tuxedos are more challenging to track down than suits, but if you've got your heart set on a tux, it is an option. Prodigy Uniform Company offers a vegan tuxedo jacket, which can be paired with a nice pair of black pants. Be sure to have your jacket in hand when you pick out your slacks to ensure the shades of black match.

Wedding Creations & Anthony's Tuxedos in Washington, DC, is a source for full vegan tuxedos for sale and rental, too.

It's not necessary to seek out tuxedos labeled "vegan" to find one that is cruelty-free. Some large retailers like Etuxedo.com carry a selection of tuxes that contain no animal products but are not categorized by the site as vegan.

Shoes

There are no rules when it comes to adorning one's feet on their wedding day. Some may want white and sparkly slippers or you can step into something bright and colorful. For those wearing a suit, you may want to match it with an oxford.

Finding vegan shoes for one's wedding need not be tedious. There are lots of options ranging from beautifully crafted selections for sale at vegan shoe stores, to synthetic styles offered by large retailers such as DSW or Zappos, to shoes ordered from the designers themselves.

Shoemaker Roni Kantor offers beautiful vegan wedding shoes in traditional styles and colors. Looks range from a simple white pump, to a slingback, to a white wedding boot. Vegan United Kingdom–based shoe designer Beyond Skin has a large number of bridal shoes available, including sandals, flats, gorgeous high heels, and shiny gold oxfords. For more traditional oxfords or a loafer to accent a suit, Brave GentleMan sells numerous high-quality styles.

And if you feel called to wear a fun bright color or something sexy and black on your feet, you can find many options at vegan shoe stores such as MooShoes, or order directly from one of the wonderful cruelty-free shoe designers such as Cri De Coeur or Olsenhaus. Of course large retailers also offer vegan shoes in a wide range of colors.

Makeup

Though not all brides will opt to wear makeup for their weddings, if you do choose to, there are a few options for ensuring your face is made up using only vegan products.

Most makeup artists will agree to work with cosmetics and tools that you provide. If you have a healthy collection of vegan makeup and brushes, this is a great option. You may pick your favorite artist (who fits your budget) and set them up with your handpicked collection of animal-free products. If you do, be sure to offer them all of your items, not just the ones you use regularly. A professional makeup artist may have some fresh ideas for colors you don't normally use. I've worked with non-vegan professional makeup artists in this way on a number of occasions and have come away with immaculate makeup. A bonus was watching them work and learning how to use my makeup in new ways.

A second option is working with a vegan makeup artist. As the vegan movement grows, vegan makeup artists are emerging around the world. The benefits of working with one include supporting a vegan in their cruelty-free business and working with someone who is thoroughly familiar with the products in his or her makeup kit. Vegan makeup artists won't be available in every geographic location, but for some of us, they are a great option.

Of course hiring a makeup artist can be costly and may be too much for one's budget to bear. Doing your own makeup for a wedding is always a possibility. If you are familiar with your face, and what looks good on it, there is nothing wrong with painting your own visage on your big day. You know your products are vegan and may be great at using them. Just remember, you'll want your makeup to be a little heavier than normal if you're having professional photographs taken. Practice your makeup in the days leading up to your wedding and take a few pictures, so that you're not experimenting hours before you tie the knot.

If you don't like makeup, if you don't want anything to do with it, that's fine, too. If your authentic self cries in the face of face paint, there's nothing wrong with a nude visage on your nuptial day.

Gifts

Weddings are a classic gift-giving event. Often, no sooner have the invitations arrived in the mail than guests start to wonder about what they will give to the couple. Of course, if we are keeping a vegan household, we may want to ask guests to only gift us with cruelty-free items. There are a few ways to encourage vegan wedding gifts. Even in receiving offerings from our guests, we can benefit animals.

Many vegans have animal advocacy organizations that we hold close to our hearts. A wedding is a wonderful occasion to request guests make a donation to one of these groups in the name of the marrying couple.

Groups we may want to consider include animal sanctuaries, shelters, and advocacy organizations. In this way, our weddings can directly benefit those who have been rescued from the cruelties of farming, breeding, or neglect.

Creating a gift registry is a great way to pre-select what items you might receive for your wedding. Most guests will stick to what a couple has picked. Registries can be created at various online retailers, so couples may choose one depending on their personal tastes and preferences. Many couples find it helpful to list items with a wide range of prices to suit the needs of guests with varying budgets.

Getting Creative

There are some other lovely ways to bring a love of animals into one's big day. Tricia Barry, a communications professional and co-owner of a winery (with her husband, Ian) worked for Farm Sanctuary at the time of her wedding. The bride and groom gave each guest a bottle of vegan wine made by Ian, decorated with charms featuring pictures of animals from the sanctuary. Meena Alagappan (who we'll meet later in this chapter) and her husband decorated the tables at their reception with centerpieces made out of stuffed toy animals, demonstrating their love for all beings.

Wedding Stories: All You Need Is Love

Many of us who find a special someone will want to make it official by getting married. And for those of us who are vegan, having a cruelty-free wedding is not only in line with our values, but reflects the loving spirit of that special day.

It's common to dream of a big wedding with a grand cake and a huge crowd. Often, in order to pay for this, we rely on a parent (or parents). If the person or people picking up the tab on your big day insist on non-vegan options against your will, you can maintain your cruelty-free baseline by paying for the wedding yourself. It's okay to mourn the grandiose nuptial day of your fantasies if you must compromise to have a vegan wedding. But won't you feel better knowing that no one suffered for you to seal the deal with the person you love?

Sometimes sticking to our vegan lifestyle means letting go of some material things—even if those physical things are related to our weddings. But letting go of the material doesn't mean compromising the joy of your wedding. And the love swells when we cut out the cruelty.

Some of us will have parents who are happy to support our vegan commitment, and some will not. Some of us will opt for a more modest affair to align our wedding with our values. Whatever the case and budget, there are many wonderful venues, clothes, cakes, and caterers that fit the plant-based bill.

I spoke to a number of women about their vegan weddings. Some were grand affairs with more than 100 guests and some were small, intimate gatherings. In each case, the bride was committed to having a cruelty-free big day, and she stuck to her values. The weddings were all joyous, loving occasions that were enjoyed by vegan and omnivore guests alike.

Inviting Guests to Join in the Compassion
Jaya Bhumitra, Animal Activist

It was their animal activism that brought Jaya Bhumitra and Christopher Locke together. The two first met at a luncheon for an animal rights organization in Los Angeles where they live. "Having veganism in common was a great bonding factor," says Jaya.

Jaya grew up in a home that included chickens as companion animals, so it was easy for her to see that they were sentient beings just as much as the family's dogs and cats. She stopped eating meat and became a vegetarian at age nine, later committing to veganism.

"I was very heavily influenced by the books I was reading," says Jaya, whose childhood library was filled with stories that featured animals either as protagonists or in important supporting roles. She says those helped her to see animals as "partners or companions rather than objects or property." As fate would have it, she married Christopher, a writer whose first book is a young adult novel called *Persimmon Takes On Humanity*, a story about a raccoon named Persimmon determined to save animals from suffering.

Upon meeting, Jaya and Christopher were quick to dive into a relationship. They reconnected soon after their initial activist lunch, attending a party together where they spent three hours talking while trying to say good night. Realizing they didn't want to say good-bye, the pair began dating. "You couldn't tear us apart once we met," says Jaya.

Jaya and Christopher's shared love of animals has always played a role in their relationship. Soon after meeting, they spent time together handing out pamphlets and working at informational tables to educate people about animal rights and veganism. When Christopher proposed to Jaya, he created a scavenger hunt for her that included the task of distributing leaflets at the Los Angeles Zoo to teach the public about cruelty to animals. In true activist form, the pair were asked to leave by the zoo's security.

A year later, in 2011, Jaya and Christopher were married in Palos Verdes, California. With veganism playing such an important role in the couple's life, they wanted their commitment to the animals featured in the celebration. They decided "Everyone should know how fabulous a vegan wedding can be," says Jaya.

Setting out to plan a cruelty-free day, "we had difficulty finding a caterer that would wow the crowd," explains Jaya, who says she and Christopher were presented with a few lackluster options during their venue search. They decided to look for a venue that would allow them to design their own menu and discovered La Venta Inn, which welcomed their ideas. "We wanted it to be very posh and demonstrate that veganism could be glamorous," says Jaya, so they selected a number of recipes from the book *The Conscious Cook* by celebrity chef Tal Ronnen to include on the menu.

The chef at La Venta Inn was "amenable and very much up to the challenge," says Jaya, adding that the venue's wedding organizer was so inspired by the couple that she went vegan herself. This was the first vegan wedding held at the inn, and the venue said it would offer Jaya and Christopher's menu to other couples looking for plant-based options.

Jaya and Christopher created a wedding website for guests with information about veganism, including a brief explanation about why it was important to them to wear vegan clothing and inviting guests to do the same for the big day. "So many people came and proudly said, 'look at my belt, look at my new wallet'—they were so excited to show us what they had purchased," says Jaya. "It wasn't mandatory, but it was thoughtful."

The food was a priority for the couple, as they considered the wedding dinner a vegan outreach opportunity. For Jaya, extravagant bridal attire was not so important. "I spent $130 on my dress," she says. "I didn't try it on until the day before the wedding, and I didn't try on my shoes until the morning of the wedding." She found her dress, made of synthetic fabric, at the website Rue La La. "I've never been that interested in clothes; for me, they're more functional," she says.

True to their love of animals, the bride and groom included a wealth of gifts for their companion animals in their wedding registry. "Our dogs are quite comfortable because of the wedding." Jaya shares that they now have dog beds in every room of their house.

Jaya and Christopher celebrated their relationship with delicious fine vegan cuisine, music that was important to them, and approximately 150 friends and family. But they also wanted to stand in solidarity with the lesbian and gay community, who could not legally marry at the time. So they waited until 2013—when same-sex marriage became legal in California—to obtain their license.

The pair received many compliments about their compassionate celebration. Says Jaya, "People were talking about the food for two years after the wedding, they so enjoyed it. We are grateful that our family and friends were so supportive of the vegan cuisine and our values."

For those considering a vegan wedding, Jaya adds, "Our compassionate beliefs are based in love. Thus, a vegan wedding is the ultimate celebration of love."

Vegan Brides Craft a Divine Day
Marie Nguyen, Airline Pilot
Olivia Nguyen, Doctor

When Canadians Olivia Nguyen and Marie Nguyen married, the only guidelines the thirty-something pair followed were those described by their hearts. Staying true to themselves, they created a wedding that reflected their own tastes and values, from the lavender-lemon vegan wedding cake to their homemade decorations.

Olivia and Marie (who shared a last name prior to marriage) had originally met as teenagers, enrolled in the same Kung Fu classes, but, "We'd never talk," says Marie. Ten years later, Olivia received a friend request from her future wife on Facebook. They soon realized their love for each other.

When Marie and Olivia first became involved romantically in 2008, Olivia was a lacto-vegetarian (consuming dairy products, but no meat or eggs). Marie was a meat-eater, "but she's very nice, so we mostly ate vegetarian food," says Olivia of their time dating. The two moved in together in 2010, around the same time that Olivia committed to veganism. They agreed to a rule of no meat in the house.

Though Marie was not vegan when the pair committed to cohabiting, she was an avid cook and easily veganized meals that she prepared for herself and Olivia. These included traditional Vietnamese dishes, made with her homemade vegan fish sauce (both women are of Vietnamese descent).

When she watched the film *Earthlings*, about animal abuses around the globe, Marie decided to stop eating meat, and eventually became completely vegan. She says, "It wasn't too hard to become vegan, because in our culture, with Buddhism, my mother used to bring me to the temple very often, and I've tried a lot of vegetarian food, which I really love." Many Buddhists adhere to a vegetarian diet.

Veganism is the couple's strongest common interest. "Actually, we're not very similar," says Olivia, "We don't like the same things at all. Like nothing. Except for food."

"We share the same love of food," adds Marie. "Let's say, when we travel, our main attraction is vegan restaurants."

In January 2015, the two decided to get married, and began planning their wedding for the approaching spring. Together, Marie and Olivia felt that a traditional Vietnamese wedding wouldn't capture their own values. Instead they expressed who they are as a couple by handcrafting the decorations, with Olivia applying her sewing skills to most of their attire. Each bride wore two ensembles, Olivia outfitted in two different dresses, while Marie donned a dress and a pants outfit. They kept their budget for clothing low, wearing uncomplicated pieces made special with Olivia's alterations. "I had it for a while and it wasn't very expensive," says Olivia of one of her dresses. "It was, say, one hundred Canadian dollars." She points out that low-priced clothes are usually vegan.

The couple held their wedding outdoors, in an apple orchard, and though they spent little on clothing and decorations, Olivia and Marie splurged on a vegan caterer. Olivia points out that "it's really hard to find a venue that allows for a caterer that you want . . . Usually they come with their own chef, and their own menu," adding, "we really like to eat, so it was important to us that the food would be good." One of the reasons the couple chose the orchard was because doing so allowed them to pick their own caterer.

A love of food, and a commitment to veganism, are important aspects of Marie and Olivia's shared life, and so they invested in excellent vegan food for their wedding. They also wanted to demonstrate for non-vegan guests how delightful plant-based cuisine can be. However, their decision to provide only cruelty-free food was met with some resistance. "It was very important to me that it was completely vegan," says Olivia, but some family members, including Marie's father, pressured the pair to offer two menus, one vegan and one not vegan. Olivia told her father-in-law, "Of course it's going to be vegan. There's no other option. Don't even try to complain."

The pair found a Montreal-based vegan caterer who prepared superb plant-based cuisine for their guests. The dishes included cucumber and rhubarb terrine and mesclun with beet sablé (a French round shortbread cookie). For dessert, they served wedding cake from Sophie Sucrée, a vegan bakery in Montreal.

Though Olivia and Marie were challenged by their family, they insisted on holding a wedding that reflected their values. They created a beautiful cruelty-free celebration at which guests dined on the finest vegan cuisine and enjoyed the couples' homegrown details.

Marie's suggestion for vegan brides planning a wedding is to "make it special and different," so that guests will have fond memories that might influence their thoughts about veganism in a positive way.

Finding Sanctuary Among Animal Friends
Christie Lee Verschoor-Schweizer, Human Resources Manager for a Wine and Spirits Company

When Christie and Robbie began dating, she was a vegetarian and "he was still an omnivore, leaning towards pescatarian," she says.

Christie, who lives in Rye, New York, had become vegetarian in approximately 2002, when she enrolled in an environmental ethics course at the college she was attending. In the class, she learned about the cruelties of factory farming and began to do her own research into the abuses animals suffer while being raised for food. "I stopped eating meat from the day that I realized what was actually happening," she says.

She and Robbie, who would become her husband, went vegan together after visiting Catskill Animal Sanctuary in 2011. The sanctuary is a spacious grassy home for rescued farm animals, located in New York's beautiful Hudson Valley. During that visit, "I was . . . enlightened and educated about what happened with the dairy and egg industries," says Christie, "and at that point, my now husband and I . . . decided together that it was time to make a change. . . . So we went vegan from that point." The couple also immediately signed up as volunteers at the sanctuary.

Robbie proposed to Christie in February 2015. When they became engaged, "Robbie first asked me what was my dream wedding. I never really dreamt of a wedding," says Christie. "My first thought was I want to get married at the Catskill Animal Sanctuary." The sanctuary is very special to Christie: "It's not just a haven for the animals, it is a haven for the people who are part of it, too." Christie explains that it helps her to be there when she's going through a rough time: "I go to the animal sanctuary and volunteer, and just be with my animal friends who don't judge you, and are so pure and kind and sweet, and support you unconditionally . . ."

Planning a small wedding, with a very supportive family, the couple didn't experience any resistance from guests about having a vegan event. "Nobody really expressed being nervous," says Christie, explaining, "My mom is vegan . . . my dad is very health conscious, so he's mostly plant-based . . ." Though no one in Robbie's family follows a vegan diet, Christie says they "realized that it's not so odd . . . that it is a moral choice that we are making and so they support it . . ."

For Christie, veganism is a very positive part of her life. "When I think of love, I think of veganism as being love. It's just pure love for all beings," she says. Those who she loves did not object to the choice for her wedding to be cruelty-free.

Held at the place that Christie had wished for, the couple were able to create their special day that honored the animals while maintaining a modest $5,000 budget. Says Christie, "It was about us, and what made us happy, and it didn't have to be this grand affair."

For food, the couple enlisted Main Course Catering in New Paltz, New York, not far from the sanctuary. Says Christie, "When they were plating the food and delivering it to our guests, it was not only delicious but it was beautiful. And so it was kind of cool for our families to see this plant-based meal which was just gorgeous and appetizing." The meal was a fantastic experience of vegan food for almost all of the guests—everyone except her meat-and-potatoes-oriented brother-in-law, who picked the seitan out of his food. For dessert, guests indulged in wedding cake prepared by local vegan bakery, Sweet Maresa's, decorated with fiddlehead ferns and small pink flowers picked from the baker's own garden.

Though Christie would only wear a vegan dress, when she began looking through photos for ideas, she didn't know what was and wasn't cruelty-free. Her mother saw one of the pictures Christie had saved and, believing it was the perfect dress for her daughter, tracked it down to a London boutique. It turned out to be made of polyester, and therefore vegan. At eighty dollars, it was just right for Christie and her budget, and her mom purchased the dress that Christie would wed in.

Out of respect for Catskill Animal Sanctuary, and the animals who live there, Christie and Robbie asked all of their guests to wear only vegan clothes to their wedding. Attendees were eager to satisfy the couple's wishes. "They were totally okay with it," says Christie. "Everyone was really sensitive about it and asked a lot of questions . . ." Clearly the pair's loved ones were not averse to making compassionate choices, and they welcomed the opportunity.

Not only were they not opposed to dressing vegan for the day, but a tour of the sanctuary inspired at least one guest to make more permanent changes. "Robbie's mom . . . said afterwards that she's not going to be able to eat pork anymore . . . once she heard on the tour about gestation crates, and the intelligence of our pig friends," says Christie.

In lieu of physical gifts, the couple requested donations be made to the sanctuary, which came to total almost $5,000. In a very real way, their love for each other led to the support and care of many rescued farm animals.

With a bouquet of succulents in hand, and wearing her own vegan makeup, Christie walked down the aisle to marry Robbie, with two of their favorite steers as witnesses. The roosters were crowing, and the turkeys gobble gobbling as the couple spoke their vows.

Meeting Online and Coming Together in Compassion
Lauren Moretti, Teacher and Graphic Designer

Lauren and her now-husband, Dan, met via the Internet in July 2003. Dan had found her by searching a website's member profiles for "Bob Dylan." When they connected in person for the first time, almost a year later, their first date was a Dylan concert.

Lauren explains that she had stopped eating meat at age fourteen, "because of Lisa Simpson," the beloved vegetarian character on animated television series, *The Simpsons.*

When her nineteenth birthday arrived, Lauren requested that instead of giving her gifts, her family watch the video *Meet Your Meat* with her, a short film about the intense suffering of animals who are farmed for food. "I was just sobbing and sobbing," says Lauren. She immediately went vegan.

Already in touch with, but not having yet met Dan when she saw the film, the two committed to veganism at the same time. When they finally connected in person, they were a cruelty-free couple.

In 2013, Lauren proposed to Dan. "I illustrated a book of our relationship, and then I gave it to him, as a proposal." They were married the following year.

Because both were committed vegans at the time they became engaged, having a vegan wedding was an easy decision for Dan and Lauren. Once Lauren made it clear that no animals or animal products would be served at her wedding, she met with no conflict, and her entire family was supportive.

The wedding was held in Cape Cod, Massachusetts, on the grounds of a house the couple rented for the week. A thread of beautiful simplicity ran throughout the event, from Lauren's cotton and lace dress to the barn-like building where they held the reception. The wedding was "really relaxed," says Lauren. "We played volleyball at the reception."

Lauren and Dan's total budget for the wedding was approximately $20,000, with about half of that spent on the house rental.

The wedding was "definitely nondenominational, it wasn't religious for sure," says Lauren, but it was spiritual in nature, with the couple married by a "life celebrant." Bringing attendees together in the spirit of the union, the approximately fifty guests were invited to each paint a stone with a good wish for the couple during the ceremony.

The reception was held in a rustic dance hall that Lauren likens to a barn, with beautiful wooden rafters and delicate white lights.

To ensure that the food was plant-based, Lauren and Dan enlisted the catering services of Boston-area vegan-friendly restaurant The Red Lentil. Dishes served included gobi Manchurian (a combination of cauliflower, chickpea flour, and tomato sauce) and a Mexican pizza that featured corn and mango. "Everyone was just blown away by the food," says Lauren. She adds that in the years following the wedding, her mother has continued to mention how good the meal was.

Opting out of a traditional gown from a bridal store, Lauren purchased a very simple vegan dress on the Etsy website.

Wanting all gifts to be cruelty-free, the couple created a small registry of items such as tea towels that they picked out online. They also accepted donations from guests toward the renovation of a house they had recently purchased. Successfully steering friends and family in a compassionate direction, the couple avoided receiving any non-vegan gifts.

Lauren explains that she and her husband's veganism is an important part of their relationship: "I don't know that I could be with somebody who wasn't vegan," she says. "I don't think I could identify with somebody who was a meat-eater, or even vegetarian, really. That is a huge part of who we are. We talk about it a lot." She adds, "We have a lot of other things in common as well, but that's a huge one for me."

Lauren encourages vegan brides-to-be to stay true to what's important to them: "If somebody were paying for my wedding, and they said there needed to be meat options, then I would not want them paying for my wedding. You know, don't compromise your values just because somebody is willing to pay for something. It's not worth it."

A Hindu-Jewish Wedding Embraces Love for All Beings
Meena Alagappan, Executive Director of a Nonprofit Humane Education Organization

Meena Alagappan didn't mull over whether she would marry Robert. When they began dating, she says, "I just knew . . . it really didn't even feel like a decision."

When Meena, who lives in New York City, started seeing Robert in July 2006, they were already both vegan. "It's funny," says Meena, ". . . we both had similar paths. He had turned vegetarian about the same time I had turned vegetarian, before I even knew him, and he became vegan about a year before me." They met while both serving on the New York City Bar's Animal Law Committee, a group that takes on legal, regulatory, and policy issues affecting animals.

Though Meena didn't fall in love with Robert because he was vegan, it represented a part of who he was that was important to her. "I think his being vegan was so consistent with so many other aspects of his personality. He was very compassionate and that was really important to me."

Both living a cruelty-free lifestyle and involved in animal causes, when Meena and Robert decided to get married, they chose to have an all-vegan wedding. Though their relatives are not vegan, "Our families totally get it, and they respect it." The couple received no complaints or criticisms for their choice.

Married in March 2007, Robert and Meena kept the wedding simple but elegant, holding it in a townhouse with approximately eighty friends and family in attendance. "We just wanted something really meaningful with close friends," says Meena, who describes the house where they held their nuptials as "quite magical . . . with beautiful sculptures and paintings . . . and a lovely garden room." Because the couple tied the knot during the venue's "off-season," the rental fee was waived, and the pair paid about $100 per person for food and drinks.

Excited about the venue they had picked, Meena and Robert encountered a small bump in the road when they attended the tasting to sample food that might be served at their reception. Though the caterer had plentiful plant-based hors d'oeuvres, the couple found their vegan entrées to be less than impressive. At the tasting, "There were a number of other couples, and they were getting these elaborate meals," says Meena. "We just got bland veggies stuck on a plate." The bride and groom were determined to serve delicious and sophisticated vegan food at their wedding, and so they approached their friend, Joy Pierson of the Candle restaurants (who we met in chapter 5), asking if the wedding caterer could use one of her recipes. With Joy's permission, the venue chef prepared Candle Cafe's popular seitan piccata, and the result was success. On the day of their wedding, guests were offered a variety of vegan starters including curried vegetable turnovers, followed by the delicious seitan dish, and a pasta option. The wedding cake was a combination of vanilla and Oreo flavored layers, created by the Vegan Treats bakery in Bethlehem, Pennsylvania.

The wedding intermingled Meena's Hindu and Robert's Jewish religious backgrounds, with the pair married by both a Hindu priest and a Jewish rabbi (who happened to be a vegetarian). For the Hindu portion of the wedding, a ritual offering of grains, milk, and flowers used a soy alternative instead of the traditional cow's milk.

For the ceremony, Meena wore a wedding saree, the traditional Indian dress for the occasion. Usually made of silk, her mother had set out to find a vegan one in India. "It was no easy feat. The saree is about six yards on average of material, and usually the ones for weddings are made out of silk," says Meena. Her mother prevailed, and Meena donned a beautiful embroidered pink saree, changing into a lengha (another traditional Indian ensemble) for the reception.

Robert and Meena offered guests no directives regarding gifts, but didn't receive anything that wasn't vegan. Meena attributes this to the intimacy of the gathering, which included only their closest friends and family. "They all knew us so well," she says. In addition to offering some useful items, guests gave donations to a farm animal sanctuary where Robert had volunteered, and some donated to the humane education organization that Meena works for.

With the union of two animal lovers, the marriage meant blending the couple's two cats and two dogs. "We were a little bit like the Brady Bunch getting together," says Meena.

Meena assures vegan brides-to-be, "It's not difficult to have your wedding be consistent with your values in every way." Though many of the couple's friends and family weren't vegan, the bride and groom stood by their beliefs for their big day, and the result was a joyful celebration that intermingled their spiritual traditions and involved no cruelty to animals.

Growing Her Own Bouquet and Planting Seeds of Love
Kirsti Gholson, Animal Activist and Singer-Songwriter

Kirsti Gholson, who lives in Woodstock, New York, was inspired to go vegan in the late 1980s, long before there were gourmet vegan cheeses or the multitude of fine plant-based restaurants that exist today. After reading an excerpt from John Robbins's book, *Diet for a New America*, a groundbreaking work about veganism, Kirsti quickly committed to a cruelty-free lifestyle. The fact that veganism wasn't popular at the time, and pre-prepared plant-based foods weren't readily available, didn't deter her.

The portion of the book that Kirsti read revealed the suffering of cows who are separated from their calves in the milk industry, and the horrible conditions that chickens farmed for their eggs are kept in. Though grocery stores and restaurants offered few vegan options at the time (other than beans, rice, pasta, and produce), Kirsti was unwavering in her ethical commitment. "If you hear this information, then there's only one thing to do, and it's not to eat animal products anymore," she says.

Immediately changing her diet, Kirsti felt spiritually unburdened. "Just realizing I could look at animals . . . and I wasn't responsible for that suffering . . . I always feel lighter, even when I'm confronted with cruelty now. There's this, *oh my gosh, I don't participate in that,* and that's huge because there is so much cruelty in the world . . ."

When Kirsti met Chris in 1999, he was a leather jacket-wearing omnivore, but she says, "I had this really powerful feeling that I'm going to be with this person . . . we really hit it off and we were practically living together right away . . ."

Chris and Kirsti were soon spending most of their time in each other's homes. Kirsti never pressured Chris to make changes to his own lifestyle, only speaking about veganism from her own perspective of being passionate about the issues. Chris was inspired, not pushed by Kirsti's commitment, and volunteered to stick with a cruelty-free lifestyle in both of their homes.

Then one day, says Kirsti, "He called me from the road and told me, 'I just want you to know it's been five days that I've been vegan.'" Today Chris works to promote veganism in the field of venture capital, traveling the world and working with companies that are disrupting the animal agriculture industry. Says Kirsti, "I'm grateful for my intuition, or I might have written him off!"

The two were married in 2002. At the time they were staying with Chris's mother on land she owned in Pennsylvania, while they helped her to renovate, and it seemed like an ideal location. The couple decided to hold their vegan wedding there. Says Kirsti, "It's a beautiful farm, not a working farm, so we just thought let's stay here and get married at the top of the hill, and overlook the valley, and make it very homegrown." They worked hard to fix up the property before the wedding and grew their own flowers for the celebration.

Though they literally found a venue in their backyard, securing a vegan caterer in the very early twenty-first century was not as easy. The farm was far away from any urban centers, so Kirsti and Chris looked to surrounding areas for possible providers of food. They found a café they liked that wasn't vegan, but was willing and excited to create a plant-based menu.

Finding a caterer was challenging, but locating a baker for a vegan wedding cake proved close to impossible. So the couple decided to take the matter into their own hands. The cake became a family project, with Kirsti and a number of Chris's close relatives pitching in to bake sheets of the vegan cake that would serve approximately 150 guests.

The bride only spent $600 on her custom-made cruelty-free wedding dress. At the time of her engagement, she worked for a textile manufacturer. One of Kirsti's favorite fabrics of his was unfortunately made of silk. So as a gift for the bride-to-be, her employer created a special vegan version of it. Kirsti then went to a dress designer, who crafted her wedding gown using the unique material.

The entire wedding had an earthy quality to it, from the bridal bouquet grown on the property, to Kirsti's sandals, which she had previously worn to her sister's wedding, to the community created cake.

The officiant asked the bride and groom to create a contract that they would sign, detailing their practical, physical, emotional, and spiritual promises and expectations in the marriage. Says Kirsti, "We agreed about our veganism, and that it's spiritual, it's the spiritual core of our life, it's not a diet, it's how we want to be and we want that compassion in the world, and with each other." So the couple put in their nuptial contract that, along with not tolerating physical or emotional abuse, neither would expect the other to live with a non-vegan. "You can't work around someone being cruel to you, or if they're being cruel to animals," says Kirsti.

Weaving the couple's love and commitment to animals into the ceremony, the officiant blessed them with words written by Chris and Kirsti: "May this marriage keep compassion for all living things strong in your hearts, and in your actions."

Kirsti and Chris heard no complaints from guests about their vegan wedding. "Everyone was supportive," says Kirsti. "They would be shocked if we were not having a vegan wedding."

Toward the end of the ceremony, a passage was read from *The Food Revolution*, another book by John Robbins, which brought up to date his *Diet for a New America*. The excerpt closes with, "It always matters how you treat other people, how you treat animals, and how you treat yourself. It always matters what you do. It always matters what you say. And it always matters what you eat."

Wedding Tips: Planning Your Vegan Nuptial Celebration

The Venue: If your venue has an attached caterer, be sure you are happy with the food prepared for your tasting. If they aren't impressing you with their serving for two, chances are they won't do a better job when they are cooking for one hundred. If no other location will do, offer them some recipes from your favorite vegan cookbooks. Many chefs will be up for a challenge.

The Clothes: Though many of the offerings from wedding gown designers are silk (not vegan), going off the beaten path will provide you with a multitude of options. Discount and small-scale bridal boutiques usually offer synthetic dresses, and some independent designers make vegan gowns. Remember, you aren't required to wear a dress that was designed as a bridal gown. There are no rules for wedding attire, so feel free to get creative.

If a suit is more your style, there are also a number of designers creating beautiful vegan two- and three-piece ensembles in a range of textiles and prices. There are also high-quality vegan oxford and loafer-style shoes available from companies such as Brave GentleMan.

The Food: Holding a wedding at a venue with no in-house caterer? You'll find a wealth of options. If no all-vegan restaurant may be enlisted, you can work with a local eatery to develop a plant-based menu. Thai, Indian, and Mediterranean restaurants can be found in most areas, and these generally offer at least a few vegan dishes. If not, you can be a vegan ambassador and help an establishment to veganize what they already offer. Or speak with a local caterer about cooking according to recipes you provide.

The Cake: Today, unlike twenty years ago, there are many vegan bakers, some that will ship their cakes. If you'd like something local, but don't have a vegan bakery close by, check in with non-vegan bakeries in your area, which may be able to create a cruelty-free cake. If all else fails, you (or someone close to you) can bake the cake. Who wouldn't appreciate a wedding cake prepared by one of the newlyweds?

The Gifts: Registries are a great way to point guests in a cruelty-free direction. Many couples also opt to request donations be made to a favorite nonprofit that helps animals, in lieu of gifts.

Some brides I spoke with suggested setting up a gift registry even if you are requesting donations be made to an organization. Many guests will purchase a gift when giving to a nonprofit is requested. If you want to be sure those gifts are in line with your ethics, it is best to give some guidance.

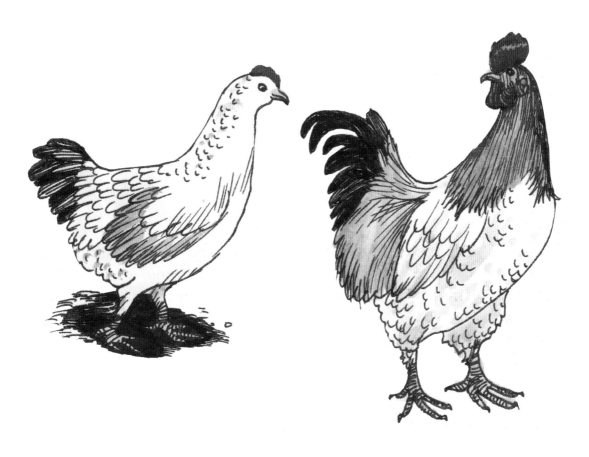

Conclusion:
Make Vegan Love, Not War

I spoke with many vegan women in the writing of this book, and each followed a unique path. Every one had arrived at their decision to eschew animal products in their own way. There was no one specific key that unlocked the door to veganism for all of them.

Just as we each may come to veganism in our own unique way, there is no formula for the perfect relationship as a vegan. Even if we are in a partnership with someone who shares our ethics concerning animals, we may disagree on other topics. However, each of us may find happiness if we are true to ourselves, and speak up for what we believe in.

I consider being vegan one of my very best qualities, and the people I know who I admire see it the same way. When I am my best self, and represent veganism in a kind, respectful, generous way, others are often drawn to me and to the vegan philosophy, whether it is someone who I am dating, or a person I meet at a dinner party. Veganism is a beautiful part of us, so why wouldn't we want to shine that light wherever we go?

If we follow our hearts to the people we connect with, let those who don't respect us fall away, and are confident in our love of animals, we are certain to find vegan love.

Resource Guide

V=All Vegan | VO=Vegan Options

Books

The 30-Day Vegan Challenge by
  Colleen Patrick-Goudreau
The China Study by T. Colin
  Campbell, PhD and Thomas M.
  Campbell II, MD
Crazy Sexy Diet by Kris Carr
Do Unto Animals by Tracey Stewart
How to be Vegan by Elizabeth
  Castoria
The Inner World of Farm Animals
  by Amy Hatkoff
Living the Farm Sanctuary Life by
  Gene Baur with Gene Stone
Main Street Vegan by Victoria
  Moran with Adair Moran
What a Fish Knows by Jonathan
  Balcombe

Caterers

Jay Astafa (V)
Location: New York, NY
www.jayastafa.com

Candle Cafe/Candle 79 (V)
Location: New York, NY
www.candle79.com

Eco Caters (VO)
Locations: Los Angeles, CA; San
  Diego, CA
www.ecocaters.com

Main Course Catering (VO)
Location: New Paltz, NY
www.maincoursecatering.com

Miss Rachel's Pantry (V)
Location: Philadelphia, PA
www.missrachelspantry.com

Sel Noir (V)
Location: Montreal, QC, Canada
www.selnoir.com

Clothing

Bead & Reel (V)
Location: Los Angeles, CA
www.beadandreel.com

Grape Cat (V)
Location: online only
www.grapecat.com

Herbivore Clothing (V)
Location: Portland, OR
www.herbivoreclothing.com

Maya Epler (V)
Location: online only
www.mayaepler.com

Vaute Couture (V)
Location: New York, NY
www.vautecouture.com

Farm Animal Sanctuaries

Catskill Animal Sanctuary
Location: Saugerties, NY
www.casanctuary.org

Farm Sanctuary
Locations: Los Angeles, CA;
   Orland, CA; Watkins Glen, NY
www.farmsanctuary.org

The Gentle Barn
Locations: Knoxville, TN; Santa
   Clarita, CA
www.gentlebarn.org

Piebird Farm Sanctuary
Location: Nipissing, ON, Canada
www.piebird.ca

Sanctuary and Safe Haven for
   Animals (SASHA) Farm
Location: Manchester, MI
www.sashafarm.org

Woodstock Farm Sanctuary
Location: High Falls, NY
www.woodstocksanctuary.org

Intimate Products

BabeLube Silicone, BabeLube
   Natural, BabeLube Silk
   lubricants (V)
www.babeland.com

Glyde Condoms (V)
www.glydeamerica.com

Sir Richard's Condoms (V)
www.sirrichards.com

Sliquid lubricant (V)
www.sliquid.com

Makeup

Arbonne (V)
www.arbonne.com

Aromi (V)
www.aromibeauty.com

Au Naturale (V)
www.aunaturalecosmetics.com

Axiology (V)
www.axiologybeauty.com

Beauty Without Cruelty (V)
www.beautywithoutcruelty.com

Blackbird Cosmetics (V)
www.blackbirdcosmetics.com

Black Moon Cosmetics (V)
www.blackmooncosmetics.com

Colorevolution (V)
www.colorevolution.com

Color Me Chad (V)
www.colormechad.com

Concrete Minerals (V)
www.concreteminerals.com

Earthly Body (V)
www.earthlybody.com

Elixery (V)
www.elixery.com

Emani (V)
www.emani.com

Everyday Minerals (V)
www.everydayminerals.com

FiOR Minerals (V)
www.fiorminerals.com

Geek Chic Cosmetics (V)
www.geekchiccosmetics.com

Glamour Dolls (V)
www.glamourdollsmakeup.com

INIKA (V)
www.inikacosmetics.com

Lime Crime (V)
www.dollskill.com

LunatiCK (V)
www.lunaticklabs.com

Modern Minerals (V)
www.modernmineralsmakeup.com

Obsessive Compulsive Cosmetics (V)
www.occmakeup.com

Overall Beauty Minerals (V)
www.overallbeauty.com

Pacifica (V)
www.pacificabeauty.com

Red Apple Lipstick (V)
www.redapplelipstick.com

Root (V)
www.rootpretty.com

Strobe Cosmetics (V)
www.strobecosmetics.com

Terre Mere Cosmetics (V)
www.terremerecosmetics.com

ZuZu Luxe (V)
www.gabrielcosmeticsinc.com/
    brand/zuzu-luxe/

Movies

Cowspiracy
www.cowspiracy.com

Earthlings
www.facebook.com/
    EarthlingsFilmOfficial

Food, Inc.
www.takepart.com

Forks Over Knives
www.forksoverknives.com

The Ghosts in Our Machine
www.theghostsinourmachine.com

Vegucated
www.getvegucated.com

Organizations

Mercy for Animals
www.mercyforanimals.org

People for the Ethical Treatment of
    Animals (PETA)
www.peta.org

Physicians Committee for
    Responsible Medicine (PCRM)
www.pcrm.org

The Vegan Society
www.vegansociety.com

Shoes and Accessories

Beyond Skin (V)
Location: available at various retailers
www.beyondskin.co.uk

Cri De Coeur (V)
Location: available at various retailers
Cridecoeur.myshopify.com

Gunas (V)
Location: available at various
    retailers
www.gunasthebrand.com

Matt & Nat (V)
Location: available at various
    retailers
www.mattandnat.com

MooShoes (V)
Locations: Los Angeles, CA; New
    York, NY
www.mooshoes.com

Websites

Girlie Girl Army
www.girliegirlarmy.com

JaneUnChained
www.janeunchained.com

The Kind Life
www.thekindlife.com

LA Fashionista Compassionista
www.lafashionistacompassionista.com

Logical Harmony
www.logicalharmony.net

Our Hen House
www.ourhenhouse.org

Vegan Beauty Review
www.veganbeautyreview.com

VegNews
www.vegnews.com

Wedding Attire

Annaborgia (V)
Location: online only
www.annaborgia.com

BHLDN (VO)
Location: available at various
    retailers
www.bhldn.com

Brave GentleMan (V)
Location: Brooklyn, NY
www.bravegentleman.com

The Cotton Bride (VO)
Location: available at various
    retailers
www.thecottonbride.com

Tara Lynn Bridal (VO)
Location: Sutton, VT
www.taralynnbridal.com

Wedding Cake Bakers

Erin McKenna's Bakery (V)
Locations: Los Angeles, CA; New
    York, NY; Orlando, FL
www.erinmckennasbakery.com

Half Baked Co. (VO)
Location: Burbank, CA
www.halfbaked.co

Sophie Sucrée (V)
Location: Montreal, QC, Canada
www.sophiesucree.com

Sweet Maresa's (V)
Location: New Paltz, NY
www.facebook.com/SweetMaresa/

Vegan Treats (V)
Location: Bethlehem, PA
www.vegantreats.com

Works Cited and Consulted

Babe. Directed by Chris Noonan. 1995.

Balcombe, Jonathan. *What a Fish Knows.* New York: Scientific American/ Farrar, Strauss and Giroux, 2016.

Baur, Gene and Gene Stone. *Living the Farm Sanctuary Life.* New York: Rodale, 2015.

Board, The Editorial. *The EPA Backs off Factory Farms.* June 14, 2013. http:// www.nytimes.com/2013/06/15/opinion/the-epa-backs-off-on-factory-farms .html?_r=1.

Born Free USA. *Slaughtered and Skinned.* http://www.bornfreeusa.org/ articles.php?more=1&p=370 (accessed 2016).

Campbell, T. Colin and Thomas M. Campbell. *The China Study.* BenBella Books, Inc., 2006.

Catanese, Christina. *Virtual Water, Real Impacts: World Water Day 2012.* March 22, 2012. https://blog.epa.gov/blog/2012/03/virtual-water-real -impacts-world-water-day-2012/.

Cats Are Different: How a Cat's Nutritional Needs are Different from a Dog's. http://www.petmd.com/cat/nutrition/evr_ct_cat_nutritional_needs_ different?page=show (accessed 2016).

Cline, Elizabeth L. *Overdressed: the shockingly high cost of cheap fashion.* New York: Portfolio/Penguin, 2012.

—. *Where Does Discarded Clothing Go?* July 18, 2014. http://www .theatlantic.com/business/archive/2014/07/where-does-discarded -clothing-go/374613/.

Coston, Susie. *To Shear or not to Shear; That is the Question (and we get it every year)*. April 28, 2009. http://www.animalsoffarmsanctuary.com/post/142910661386/to-shear-or-not-to-shear-that-is-the-question.

Cowspiracy. Directed by Kip and Keegan Kuhn Andersen. 2014.

Cruelty-Free & Vegan Brand List. http://logicalharmony.net/cruelty-free-vegan-brand-list/ (accessed 2016).

Earthlings. Directed by Shaun Monson. 2005.

Eisnitz, Gail A. *Slaughterhouse*. Prometheus Books, 2006.

Farm Sanctuary. *Factory Farming*. http://www.farmsanctuary.org/learn/factory-farming (accessed 2016).

Farm to Fridge. Directed by Lee Iovino. 2011.

Fields, JL. *Vegan Pressure Cooking: Delicious Beans, Grains, and One-Pot Meals in Minutes*. Fair Winds Press, 2015.

Forks Over Knives. Directed by Lee Fulkerson. 2011.

The Ghosts in Our Machine. Directed by Liz Marshall. 2013.

Gruber, Philip. *Avoid Manure Pits' Fatal Fumes*. August 26, 2016. http://www.lancasterfarming.com/farm_life/health_and_safety/avoid-manure-pits-fatal-fumes/article_b8f6868b-1b16–506b-a375-ab7df60afba5.html.

Gunn, Tim and Kate Moloney. *Tim Gunn: A Guide to Quality, Taste & Style*. New York: Abrams Image, 2007.

Happy Cow. *Compassionate Threads for Everyone*. https://www.happycow.net/vegtopics/fashion (accessed 2016).

Homes, Volker. *On the Scent: Conserving Musk Deer - The Uses of Musk and Europe's Role in its Trade*. TRAFFIC Europe, 1999.

Humane Society International. *About Cosmetics Animal Testing*. http://www.hsi.org/issues/becrueltyfree/facts/about_cosmetics_animal_testing.html (accessed 2016).

Humane Society of the United States. *The Welfare of Animals in the Egg Industry.* http://www.humanesociety.org/assets/pdfs/farm/welfare_egg.pdf.

Jackson, David and Gary Marx. *Spills of Pig Waste Kill Hundreds of Thousands of Fish in Illinois.* August 5, 2016. http://www.chicagotribune.com/news/watchdog/pork/ct-pig-farms-pollution-met-20160802-story.html.

Jackson, Jo. *Are Cats Carnivores.* 2016. http://pets.thenest.com/cats-carnivores-7671.html.

Food, Inc. Directed by Robert Kenner. 2008.

Malerman, Josh. *Bird Box.* Ecco, 2014.

Mercy for Animals. *Breeding Misery: Inside the Pork Industry.* http://pigs.mercyforanimals.org.

Messina, Virginia and JL Fields. *Vegan for Her: The Woman's Guide to Being Healthy and Fit on a Plant-Based Diet.* Da Capo Lifelong Books.

Moran, Victoria and Adair Moran. *Main Street Vegan.* New York: Tarcher/Penguin, 2012.

Patrick-Goudreau, Colleen. *Food for Thought podcast.* 2016.

—. *The 30-Day Vegan Challenge.* Montali Press, 2015.

People for the Ethical Treatment of Animals. *25 Vegan Candies for a "Spooktacular" Halloween.* http://www.peta.org/living/food/25-vegan-halloween-candies/ (accessed 2016).

—. *Animals Used for Clothing.* http://www.peta.org/issues/animals-used-for-clothing/.

—. *Meet Your Meat.* http://www.peta.org/videos/meet-your-meat/.

—. *Videos.* http://www.peta.org/videos/ (accessed 2016).

—. *What's Wrong With Beeswax?* http://www.peta.org/about-peta/faq/whats-wrong-with-beeswax/ (accessed 2016).

Robbins, John. *Diet for a New America*. Walpole, NH: Stillpoint, 1987.

—. *The Food Revolution*. Conari Press, 2010.

Ronnen, Tal. *The Conscious Cook*. William Morrow Cookbooks, 2009.

Rowe, Martin, ed. *Running, Eating, Thinking*. Lantern Books, 2014.

Ryan, Pam. *10 Common Cosmetic Ingredients That are Derived From Animal Products*. February 24, 2015. http://www.onegreenplanet.org/animalsandnature/common-cosmetic-ingredients-derived-from-animal-products/.

Saint Clair, Stella Rose. *How to Tell if Your Makeup is Truly Vegan*. May 14, 2013. https://www.beautylish.com/a/vxycr/how-to-tell-if-your-makeup-is-truly-vegan.

Shelley, Mary. *Frankenstein*. New York: Dover Publications, 1994.

Singer, Jasmin. *Always Too Much and Never Enough*. Berkley, 2016.

Steinfeld, Henning, et al. *Livestock's Long Shadow: Environmental Issues and Options*. Rome: Food and Agriculture Organization of the United Nations.

Stewart, Tracey. *Do Unto Animals*. New York: Artisan, 2015.

Taurine Deficiency in Cats. http://www.petmd.com/cat/conditions/cardiovascular/c_ct_taurine_deficiency (accessed 2016).

Trumps, Valerie. "Taurine: Why Cats Need It." http://www.pet360.com/cat/nutrition/taurine-why-cats-need-it/tUtlP691i0-bL_j2TW4nXw (accessed 2016).

United States Environmental Protection Agency. "Animal Feeding Operations in Region 9." *Notes from Underground*, Fall 2001.

The VegNews Guide to Vegan Candy. October 26, 2015. http://vegnews.com/articles/page.do?pageId=4487&catId=2.

Vegucated. Directed by Marisa Miller Wolfson. 2011.

We Are All Noah. Directed by Tom Regan. 1986.

Acknowledgments

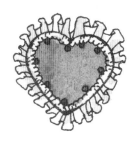

The first album by one of my favorite eighties bands, the Thompson Twins, was a record called *A Product of . . . (Participation). Vegan Love* has been, in every way, a product of participation. I have many people to thank for their help and enthusiasm.

First, I want to thank my vegan love, Dietrich Schmidt. He is my partner in life and cat-parenting, and inspired me to write on the topic of dating and partnering as a vegan.

I pursued writing *Vegan Love* in large part because of the enthusiasm of my dad, Martin Gottfried, who passed away before the book's completion. Though not vegan, and not a gal, he was excited about the book, and encouraged me to write it from the moment I shared the idea with him.

Thank you also to my mom, Jane Lahr, who cheered me on as I worked on the book, and gave me valuable feedback.

A huge thank you to my agent, Joan Brookbank, who immediately responded when I first emailed her about *Vegan Love*. She jumped on board to represent it, and sought out the perfect publisher.

There are a number of individuals to thank at Skyhorse Publishing, who went above and beyond the call of duty. I want to thank Nicole Frail, my editor, for acquiring *Vegan Love*, patiently answering all of my questions (even as they increased in frequency), and for sprinkling her editorial fairy dust on the book. Thank you also to assistant editor Leah Zarra for delving into the details to craft a better book, and for enthusiasm that was palpable throughout the process. I am also grateful for the wonderful work of cover designer Jenny Zemanek.

The illustrations created by Dame Darcy for *Vegan Love* are truly special, and it would not be the same book without her incredible contribution. A huge thank you to her for creating visuals for the book that are so much greater than even what I'd imagined.

I want to thank the many people who let me interview them for the book, and those who so generously offered makeup tips. Thank you also to the various organizations that granted me permission to use their logos in writing about makeup: Certified Vegan, Choose Cruelty Free, Leaping Bunny, People for the Ethical Treatment of Animals, and The Vegan Society. These groups work tirelessly to assess whether various products are tested on animals or contain animal products.

Thank you to Farm Sanctuary and their president and cofounder, Gene Baur, for support, help, and wonderful quotes to include in the text. Thank you to Susie Coston, Farm Sanctuary's National Shelter Director and resident farm animal whisperer for teaching me so much about the animals, supporting my work, and allowing me to quote her. Thank you also to Sarah Lux at Farm Sanctuary for help and kindness.

An enormous thank you Charlotte Van Vlack Belsito, who helped me to transcribe the interviews included in the book. I couldn't have done it without her.

Thank you to Nancy Goldstein for such thoughtful feedback and suggestions. Thank you to Jasmin Singer for her enthusiasm about the project from day one and advice that was so helpful. Thank you to Jane Rosenman for valued input and advice early on in the process of writing the book. And to Kara Davis, for her incredible editorial eye, wisdom, love of animals, and understanding of queer concerns in reviewing the book and sharing feedback.

I am blessed to have so many friends who cheered me on as I wrote. Thank you to Elizabeth Blake, my oldest and best friend, for so much support and love. Thank you to Alexandra Jacobs for re-entering my life as a friend, and granting me a fantastic interview. Thank you to friends and neighbors Shelley Wollert and Allen Farmelo for wonderful company and valuable feedback. Thank you to Rachel Stevens for friendship, support, and being excited about my vegan shoes. Thank you to Damian Miller for always wanting to go out to a vegan lunch when in town, and asking about the book each time we met. Thank you to John Carruthers for supporting me in my writing and being curious about my ideas. Thank you to Lori Majewski, whose work I hugely respect, for being excited about this project of mine. Thank you to Luke Jenner for always cheering me on and great conversations about the creative process. Thank you to Pam Nashel Leto for fun lunches that erased any stress, if only for an hour at a time. Thank you to Katy Krassner, for being enthusiastic about my work as a writer, and for the Duran Duran DVD mentioned in the introduction.

And thank you to Aimee Christian, for being my first vegan friend, taking me to Farm Sanctuary, and opening the door for me to a compassionate lifestyle.

About the Author

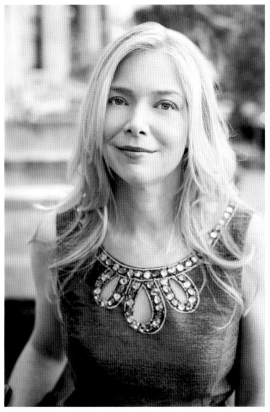

Photo credit: Jessica Mahady

Maya Gottfried (www.mayabidaya.com) is the author of several books for children, including *Good Dog* and *Our Farm: By the Animals of Farm Sanctuary*. She has also written for various online and print publications including *People* online, *Lilith Magazine*, and *The Huffington Post*. In addition to her writing she has worked extensively in the field of public relations for books, music, and animal welfare causes. She lives outside of New York City with her life partner, Dietrich Schmidt, and their three adopted cats, Lucian, Bunny, and Gandalf.